Stomach Problems: Relief At Last

Books by Vernon Coleman

The Medicine Men (1975)
Paper Doctors (1976)
Everything You Want To Know About Ageing (1976)
Stress Control (1978)
The Home Pharmacy (1980)
Aspirin or Ambulance (1980)
Face Values (1981)
Guilt (1982)
The Good Medicine Guide (1982)
Stress And Your Stomach (1983)
Bodypower (1983)
An A to Z Of Women's Problems (1984)
Bodysense (1984)
Taking Care Of Your Skin (1984)
A Guide to Child Health (1984)
Life Without Tranquillisers (1985)
Diabetes (1985)
Arthritis (1985)
Eczema and Dermatitis (1985)
The Story Of Medicine (1985, 1998)
Natural Pain Control (1986)
Mindpower (1986)
Addicts and Addictions (1986)
Dr Vernon Coleman's Guide To Alternative Medicine (1988)
Stress Management Techniques (1988)
Overcoming Stress (1988)
Know Yourself (1988)
The Health Scandal (1988)
The 20 Minute Health Check (1989)
Sex For Everyone (1989)
Mind Over Body (1989)
Eat Green Lose Weight (1990)
Why Animal Experiments Must Stop (1991)
The Drugs Myth (1992)
Why Doctors Do More Harm Than Good (1993)
Stress and Relaxation (1993)
Complete Guide to Sex (1993)
How to Conquer Backache (1993)
How to Conquer Arthritis (1993)
Betrayal of Trust (1994)
Know Your Drugs (1994, 1997)

Food for Thought (1994)
The Traditional Home Doctor (1994)
I Hope Your Penis Shrivels Up (1994)
People Watching (1995)
Relief from IBS (1995)
The Parent's Handbook (1995)
Oral Sex: Bad Taste And Hard To Swallow? (1995)
Why Is Pubic Hair Curly? (1995)
Men in Dresses (1996)
Power over Cancer (1996)
Crossdressing (1996)
How To Get The Best Out Of Prescription Drugs (1996)
How To Get The Best Out of Alternative Medicine (1996)
How To Conquer Arthritis (1996)
High Blood Pressure (1996)
How To Stop Your Doctor Killing You (1996)
How To Overcome Toxic Stress (1990, 1996, 2000)
Fighting For Animals (1996)
Alice and Other Friends (1996)
Dr Coleman's Fast Action Health Secrets (1997)
Dr Vernon Coleman's Guide to Vitamins and Minerals (1997)
Spiritpower (1997)
Other People's Problems (1998)
How To Publish Your Own Book (1999)
How To Relax and Overcome Stress (1999)
Animal Rights – Human Wrongs (1999)
Superbody (1999)
The 101 Sexiest, Craziest, Most Outrageous Agony Column Questions (and
     Answers) of All Time (1999)
Food for Thought [revised edition] (2000)
Strange but True (2000)
The Complete Guide To Life (2000)

reports
Prostate Trouble (2000)
Vitamins and Minerals (2000)
How to Campaign (2000)
Genetic Engineering (2000)
Osteoporosis (2000)
Vaccines (2000)
Alternative Medicine (2000)

novels
The Village Cricket Tour (1990)
The Man Who Inherited a Golf Course (1995)
The Bilbury Chronicles (1992)
Bilbury Grange (1993)
Mrs Caldicot's Cabbage War (1993)
Bilbury Revels (1994)
Deadline (1994)
Bilbury Country (1996)
Second Innings (1999)
Around the Wicket (2000)

short stories
Bilbury Pie (1995)

on cricket
Thomas Winsden's Cricketing Almanack (1983)
Diary Of A Cricket Lover (1984)

as Edward Vernon
Practice Makes Perfect (1977)
Practise What You Preach (1978)
Getting Into Practice (1979)
Aphrodisiacs – An Owner's Manual (1983)
Aphrodisiacs – An Owner's Manual (Turbo Edition) (1984)
The Complete Guide To Life (1984)

as Marc Charbonnier
Tunnel (novel 1980)

with Alice
Alice's Diary (1989)
Alice's Adventures (1992)

with Dr Alan C Turin
No More Headaches (1981)

Stomach Problems: Relief At Last

How You Can Conquer Wind,
Belching, Flatulence, Indigestion,
Heartburn, Gastritis, Ulcers And Other
Similar Digestive Problems

Vernon Coleman

European Medical Journal

Publishing in 2000 by the European Medical Journal Books, Publishing House, Trinity Place, Barnstaple, Devon EX32 9HJ England

Previous publishing history: Part of this book was first published in the UK by Sheldon Press, under the title *Stress and your Stomach* in 1982.

ISBN: 1 898947 74 0

A catalogue record for this book is available from the British Library.

Printed and bound by: Antony Rowe Limited, Wiltshire

Note
All case histories in this book have been changed to protect the identity and confidentiality of the individuals concerned. Any likenesses to human beings, living or dead, are purely coincidental.

Warning
This book is not intended to be, and cannot be, an alternative to personal, professional, medical advice.

Readers should immediately consult a trained and properly qualified health professional, whom they trust and respect, for advice about any symptom or health problem which requires diagnosis, treatment or any kind of medical attention.

While the advice and information in this book are believed to be accurate at the time of going to press, neither the author nor the publisher can accept any legal responsibility for errors or omissions which may be made.

Dedicated to Donna Antoinette Coleman and Brian Stockwell; golfers with stout digestions.

CONTENTS

INTRODUCTION

'I am convinced digestion is the great secret of life,' wrote the legendary English essayist, wit and clergyman Sydney Smith in a letter to Arthur Kinglake.

Sydney Smith was writing at the start of the 19th century but his comment is probably truer today than ever before.

Digestive problems are so common that I doubt if there are many individuals over the age of thirty who can claim that they've never had any problems with this part of their body. Indigestion, heartburn, wind and other, similar problems are so common as to be unremarkable. And all the evidence suggests that problems of this type are destined to continue to get commoner and commoner.

The two main causes of problems affecting the stomach are diet and stress. Most of us eat a diet which is pretty well guaranteed to cause stomach problems. And most of us are constantly under too much stress.

Most of us have a weak point. Some people get headaches when they are under pressure. Others get asthma, heart pains, diarrhoea or skin rashes. And millions get stomach problems.

The human body, like most complex pieces of machinery doesn't go all wrong at once. There is usually one part that is weaker than the rest.

If you are a regular sufferer from indigestion, ulcer pains

or other stomach symptoms then the chances are that your stomach is your weak point. Make sure you see your doctor and tell him all your symptoms.

It is often extremely difficult for the individual who has digestive symptoms to know precisely how serious the problem is.

I have known some patients with quite severe peptic ulceration complain of nothing more than intermittent mild pain, while on the other hand I have also known patients complain of very bad pain when subsequent investigations have shown no evidence whatsoever of there being any physical signs of damage.

(It is also by no means always easy to be certain about the diagnosis when dealing with chest pain. In all sorts of patients, but particularly in men in their thirties, forties and fifties, early heart pain may occasionally mimic bad indigestion and a mistaken diagnosis at this stage can prove fatal.)

To be sure about the diagnosis you must consult a qualified and competent doctor in whom you have faith and whom you trust before you try to treat yourself. I suggest that you should visit your doctor if you have had any recurring pains which you suspect might be due to stomach problems, or if you have any pain which persists for more than five days. Obviously, you should visit your doctor anyway if you vomit up blood, if you have severe pain or if you notice any other symptoms such as weight or appetite loss.

One of the most important things that your doctor can do is to confirm the diagnosis or exclude any serious pathology. But most doctors will also offer some form of treatment.

Not long ago the routine for patients complaining of indigestion type pains followed a pretty certain pattern. To begin with patients would be given a prescription for an antacid remedy and told to cut out tobacco and alcohol and to stick to a milky diet. Plenty of fish and milky rice pudding was usually recommended.

If this routine didn't work the patient would probably be sent along to the hospital to have a barium meal examination. And if the barium meal examination showed the existence of a peptic ulcer the patient would probably be sent along to see a surgeon who would simply chop out the affected piece of intestinal tract.

Today the surgical approach is rarely considered until other options have been explored. And the most popular option is to prescribe one of the growing number of drugs sold specifically to help 'heal' an ulcer.

Many treatments will help relieve your symptoms and they may even temporarily speed up the natural healing process. But what you must remember is that taking drugs to help cure indigestion (or any other stomach problem) can only offer a short-term solution. If your car has a leaky radiator hose you can solve the problem temporarily by pouring more water into the radiator. This will not, however, provide a lasting answer to your problem. If you have a leak in the roof you can disguise the damp patch on the bedroom ceiling by re-papering every week, but that won't stop the damp patch reappearing the next time it rains.

Your stomach problems may well be relieved temporarily by the use of an antacid or one of the new 'wonder' drugs recommended for patients with stomach problems. But if the cause of your problem remains unchanged then the chances are high that your symptoms will eventually recur.

This book is not intended to take the place of a doctor. It would be absurd and dangerous for any doctor to try to offer individual clinical advice without a personal consultation.

If you have a persistent or recurrent digestive problem then you must see your doctor. It would be reckless and foolhardy for either of us to imagine that a book could possibly replace a face to face consultation and a proper physical examination.

I have, therefore, deliberately not included any information about the drugs which are available for the treatment of stomach problems. If you need to take medicines then you need to see a doctor. What I have done is to pack this book with advice and information designed to help you keep your stomach healthy or to restore it to good health if problems have already developed in that area. The aim of this book is to explain why your problem developed in the first place. And, much more important, how you can best ensure that it goes away and doesn't come back again.

Vernon Coleman, Devon 2000

PART ONE:

MEET YOUR STOMACH: THE BATTLE-GROUND

There was a time when all the body's members
Rebell'd against the belly; thus accus'd it:
That only like a gulf it did remain
I' th' midst o' th' body, idle and unactive,
Still cupboarding the viand, never bearing
Like labour with the rest; where th' other instruments
Did see and hear, devise, instruct, walk, feel
And, mutually participate, did minister
Unto the appetite and affection common
Of the whole body. The belly answered
'True is it, my incorporate friends,' quoth he,
'That I receive the general food at first
Which you do live upon; and fit it is,
Because I am the storehouse and the shop
Of the whole body. But, if you do remember,
I send it through the rivers of your blood
Even to the court, the heart, to th' seat o' th' brain,
And, through the cranks and offices of man,
The strongest nerves and small inferior veins
From me receive that natural competency
Whereby they live.'

WILLIAM SHAKESPEARE (1564-1616), CORIOLANUS

19

The intestinal or alimentary tract has the simple function of making food supplies available to the body and allowing the unwanted surplus to be discharged at the distant end of the tract. Since the whole system is basically a rather long tube it is quite reasonable to argue that food passing through the alimentary tract isn't actually inside the body at all until it has been absorbed through the intestinal wall at some point.

An average sort of intestinal tract in an average sort of adult will be about 9 metres (30 feet) long. Those 9 metres of gut are divided into a number of different parts. Each part of the intestinal tract has its own job to do.

The first part of the tube is called the oesophagus or gullet and this does nothing more than simply carry food directly from the mouth to the stomach. The stomach is dilated in comparison to the rest of the tract and, depending on your fancy, either looks a bit like one of those leather drinking bottles that nomads carry with them through the desert or resembles a small, slightly misshapen hot water bottle.

It is the job of your stomach to turn the vast variety of assorted foods that you drop into it into a moveable thick soup which can be passed on into the next part of your intestinal tract. The stomach is a vestibule to the rest of the intestinal tract and it is here that food is prepared for digestion. The stomach, it is important to understand, is not just a passive repository for food.

Your stomach helps digest food in two ways. First the cells of the stomach lining produce something like three litres of gastric juice every day. Of the different substances which make up these juices probably the most important is hydrochloric acid which is produced by the parietal cells. These exist in the stomach wall in a total population of something approaching a billion.

The power and effect of these juices is enhanced by the stomach's muscular wall which churns the food and the juices together before squirting the resultant soup-like mixture through a valve into the next part of the intestinal tract, the duodenum.

It is these two properties of the stomach which give it its power as a digestive force and there are a number of different factors which can influence both the production of acid and the activity of the stomach's muscular wall. Of these factors the two which are of the greatest significance in the normal stomach are the presence and absence of food.

A good deal of research has been done over the years to show just how food can trigger off the production of acid and the start of the digestive process. It is known that there are special cells in the stomach lining which can be triggered by the presence of food to produce a hormone which then stimulates the production of acid. And it is known that when the stomach is stretched by the presence of food yet another complex reflex mechanism is triggered off in such a way as to produce more acid.

Within an hour or two after a meal has been eaten the stomach will be empty and the partly digested food will have been passed on through a fairly narrow opening into the duodenum. The opening which divides the stomach from the duodenum is guarded by a muscular valve called the pyloric sphincter which only opens when food is ready to move on out of the stomach.

By the time food gets into the duodenum it will have been attacked by the enzymes in both human saliva and the stomach's own digestive juices. In the duodenum it is met by bile which is produced by the liver and which helps digest fat, and by the enzymes which are produced by the pancreas to help break down proteins, fats and starch.

The more or less completely digested food is now passed on into the small intestine where another set of enzymes completes the digestive process and where the resultant tiny particles are absorbed into the wall of the intestine.

By the time food has got to the end of the small intestine and is about to enter the part of the intestinal tract known as the large bowel it is little more than waste residue. Water is removed in the colon and mucus is secreted to help the stools pass easily along to the exit point.

PART TWO

WHY WE GET PROBLEMS

'I lead a most dyspeptic, solitary, self shrouded life: consuming, if possible in silence, my considerable daily allotment of pain.'
THOMAS CARLYLE, IN A LETTER TO RALPH WALDO EMERSON,
FEBRUARY 8TH 1839

Introduction

The normal functioning of the stomach (and, indeed, the intestinal tract as a whole) depends largely on there being a good, steady supply of the right sort of food. The stomach's only function is to prepare food for digestion and if there is too little or too much of the wrong sort of food then the stomach will begin to exhibit signs of distress.

There is some evidence which suggests that stomach and duodenal problems run in families and that men are more likely to get duodenal trouble than women. But genetics plays only a small part in the development of stomach disorders. And taking care about what you put into your stomach can decide whether the genetic factor really does play a significant role in your future health.

The other big factor which decides whether or not you develop a stomach problem is the amount of stress you are exposed to – and how well you deal with that stress.

Research workers are still not absolutely certain about precisely what other problems can cause damage to the stomach, but there is considerable evidence to suggest that drinking too much alcohol, smoking too many cigarettes and taking too many of the wrong sort of drugs will all produce damage to the digestive part of the intestinal tract by affecting the rate at which acid is produced, the speed and nature of the movements of the stomach's muscle wall, or the stomach lining.

Learn to think of the first signs of stomach trouble as early warning signs. If you suffer from heartburn, indigestion or wind then your body is simply passing on a message. You're pushing too hard and your stomach cannot stand the pace. Try and decide exactly what it is that is putting you under excessive pressure and try and decide how best to cope. You may need to cut back your exposure to stress or you may need to build up your own capacity to withstand stress.

We Put The Wrong Things In Our Stomachs (And Eat Them Too Quickly)

Just about everything about the way we eat has changed dramatically during the last century or so.

Although those of us in the 'developed' world now have access to more food – and more varieties of food – that doesn't necessarily mean that we eat better or more wisely.

Most of us eat the wrong foods and we eat far too many of them.

But not all our troublesome eating habits are new.

We eat at the wrong times and at the wrong speed but Robert Louis Stevenson knew all about that hazard when he wrote: 'He sows hurry and reaps indigestion' in *Virginibus Puerisque*.

We eat in a hurry so that we can get back to work. We eat

while we are working. We eat while we are travelling. We eat overcooked fast food which consists of little but fat and additives. We eat pre-packaged foods which are rich in fat and chemicals. We eat foods which are packed with drugs and hormones – some of which cause cancer. We drink too much alcohol, too many sugar rich drinks and too much caffeine. We drink far too little fresh water.

It is, perhaps, hardly surprising that stomach problems are now endemic in our modern society.

We Expose Ourselves To Too Much Stress

The other important factor in the development of stomach and duodenal problems is stress. I believe that the evidence which exists is convincing.

Although the subject of stress has been discussed in a great many different magazines and newspapers over the years there are still many misconceptions about precisely what stress is and what sort of people suffer from it.

Even the very word 'stress' is the subject of much confusion, for some people use it to describe the sort of activity, pressure and strain that cause mental anguish and physical damage, while others use it as a general term to describe the physiological response to pressure. In this book I have used the word stress to refer to the sort of pressures that cause problems rather than the physical and mental problems themselves. I have used the phrase 'stress-induced disease' to refer to disorders produced by stress.

WHO SUFFERS FROM STRESS?

If you asked the average man or woman in the street to describe the sort of individual he thought might be most likely to suffer from too much stress he would probably mention taxi-drivers, airline pilots, air traffic controllers and business executives. Indeed I suspect that some people imagine that stress is something endured almost exclusively by harassed businessmen rushing from airport to airport, clutching briefcases stuffed to the twin brass combination locks with documents and contracts.

In practice, of course, it is quite impossible to classify stress sufferers by occupation or by any other criterion. The simple truth is that anyone can suffer from too much stress and it is the individual's susceptibility to stress rather than the extent of the stress which governs the amount of damage that is done.

Some people are extremely vulnerable to stress and they will suffer a good deal from a fairly minimal amount of pressure. Other individuals, in contrast, are capable of withstanding enormous pressures without suffering any ill-effects at all and may indeed seem to thrive as the pressure builds up. This is not, of course, a phenomenon which is peculiar to stress. It is just as true to say that some people are more susceptible than others to colds.

Nevertheless, despite the fact that there is a good deal of individual variation in susceptibility to stress it is a fact that there are some situations and some pressures which are particularly likely to produce stress-induced disease. These situations and pressures are rarely connected to individual occupations but are more general, and can as easily affect a nurse or a shop assistant, as a company director or high-level business executive.

HOW DOES STRESS CAUSE SYMPTOMS?

Built into your body there is a remarkable series of defence mechanisms designed to enable you to deal with threats and dangers as quickly and as effectively as possible. The aim of these mechanisms is simply to enable you to defend yourself and to survive whatever the threat may be.

These defence mechanisms have been developed and improved over very many centuries and they are primarily designed to cope with immediate problems requiring urgent action.

If, for example, you're about to be attacked by a man-eating sabre-toothed tiger then your body will automatically prepare for the attack.

Information about the impending attack will be fed immediately into your central nervous system and the pituitary gland deep inside your skull will produce a hormone called adrenocorticotrophic hormone (ACTH) which is designed specifically to stimulate the adrenal glands. The adrenal glands in turn then produce two sets of hormones: adrenaline and steroids. These hormones from the adrenal gland have an effect throughout the body. They increase the blood pressure, close down the superficial blood vessels, improve the blood supply to the muscles, tense the muscles and even make your hairs stand on end. And they increase the flow of acid into your stomach.

All these actions have a purpose. Your blood pressure goes up and your heart rate increases so that your muscles and brain have the best possible supply of nutrients. Your muscles tense so that you are ready to spring into action. Your superficial blood vessels constrict so that the amount of blood circulating through the skin is kept to a minimum. This not only ensures that there is a good supply to the essential organs, but it also limits the amount of blood that will be lost if you are bitten by the tiger. Your hairs stand on end to try and make you look larger. The extra acid that flows into your stomach is designed to turn any food there into digestible form just as soon as possible. Your body needs all the energy supply it can get its hands on!

Now if you *really* are being threatened by a sabre-toothed tiger all these actions are a tremendous help, of course. Your body will be that much better able to cope as a result of all these changes. You'll be able to run faster, jump higher and punch harder. You'll be much more likely to survive the attack thanks to the flood of hormones that have swept through your body.

But, unfortunately, the human body cannot differentiate between stressful situations, and it has not yet learned to adapt to our modern way of life in which problems are not usually so easily solved by simple physical methods.

What happens, therefore, is that when you are threatened with problems such as redundancy or a retirement that you don't really want to take, your body will react in exactly the same way that it would have reacted to that sabre-toothed tiger. There will be changes in your cardiovascular system and your blood pressure will rise. There will be a continuing flood of acid into your stomach and you may also develop a peptic ulcer as a souvenir of the experience.

Whereas the confrontation with the tiger would have been over one way or another quite quickly, the state of unemployment (or whatever stress it is that you are facing) may well go on for weeks, months or even years. And the result of that is that your body's own defence system, designed to help you cope more effectively with danger, is in fact likely to produce problems of its own.

The human body is still designed for operation in environments where action must be taken quickly and where stimuli are unlikely to go on for too long. It has not yet adapted properly to modern life where stimuli are likely to persist and where there is often no escape from those stimuli.

WOLF'S STUDIES

One of the most dramatic studies to deal with the effect of stress on the stomach was done by Dr Stewart Wolf. Dr Wolf's work was largely done with the acid of a man who is simply known in the medical literature as Tom.

When he was a mere nine years old Tom made the mistake of stuffing some scalding hot clam chowder into his mouth. The scalding substance burned his oesophagus so badly that the tube became sealed and Tom could no longer eat by swallowing food in the normal way. An opening had to be made in his abdominal wall for food to be put directly into the stomach.

As the years went by Tom adapted very well to this problem and would chew his food in his mouth before spitting it into a funnel leading in through his abdominal wall. He adapted so well, in fact, that he deliberately kept away from doctors and it was more or less by chance that he and Dr Wolf ever met.

When they did meet, however, Dr Wolf and the doctor with whom he was working (who by one of those strange coincidences happened to be called Dr Wolff), arranged for Tom to be given a job as a hospital orderly. Over the following years they wrote a number of scientific papers about Tom and his stomach, many of which are still regarded as of great significance. One of their most important discoveries was that the lining to Tom's stomach could be affected not just by food but also by stress.

They discovered that if Tom was annoyed or angry then his stomach wall cells produced huge amounts of unnecessary acid in just the same way as the skin on his face would go bright red. And they also discovered that when Tom was angry and his stomach was producing too much acid they could reverse the whole process by helping to reassure and calm him.

From what we know about the way in which stress prepares the human body for action by pushing up the rate at which the circulatory system carries oxygen and food to the muscles it seems likely that the extra burst of acid is designed to ensure that any food supplies still awaiting the digestive problem will be prepared for absorption into the body as rapidly as possible.

Now although this piece of evidence seems fairly convincing, and although I and many other doctors have met and dealt with a huge number of patients whose stomach and duodenal problems can be linked directly to stress, there still isn't any conclusive evidence that stress causes stomach problems.

And I'm afraid that there isn't likely to ever be any conclusive evidence linking stress and stomach disease for the very simple reason that it is almost impossible to measure the amount of stress that individuals are under and it is impossible to measure the amount of stress that individuals were under when they first started to develop their stomach problems. Establishing a strict and formal relationship between stress and stomach problems is made even more difficult by the fact that individuals who are under stress are very often also the same sort of people who drink too much alcohol, smoke too much and eat irregularly or too quickly. (I believe that stress is very often the underlying cause for many of these habits too but I can't prove that either.)

However, my own experience when I was a family doctor suggests that the vast majority of stomach and duodenal problems are either caused directly by stress or are exacerbated by it.

WHAT CAUSES STRESS?

It isn't possible to list all the different stresses and strains which can cause damage. But on the following pages I have tried to describe some of the types of stress most likely to produce problems. In particular, I have tried to suggest some of the less obvious ways in which we can all find ourselves under pressure.

These sources of distress are included in this book simply as an introduction to the subject. I have changed all the names and details of the patients whose case histories I have used so that they are completely unrecognisable. Most readers could undoubtedly add many more sources of stress to the list.

Ways to deal with these pressures and the pains they produce are discussed later in this book.

The pressure to achieve: Robert Smith

The pressure to achieve starts very early these days. The youngest patient I ever saw with indigestion was just eight years old and he had acquired his gastro-intestinal symptoms simply because his parents and schoolteachers had put him under too much pressure.

From the age of six, Robert Smith was expected to do at least an hour's homework every evening and at the weekends he was shut into his bedroom for at least two hours every Saturday and Sunday. The pressure on young Robert to do well in all his academic subjects was matched only by the pressure on him to do well at sports. When he wasn't studying Robert was kept busy with extra coaching in cricket, football and athletics. The aim was clearly not to take part but to win. Robert was encouraged to keep a poster in his bedroom recording his athletic achievements .

All this was just too much, and when he was eight years old Robert began to complain of regular symptoms of indigestion. Investigations showed that there was no sign of any peptic ulceration, but there was little doubt in the mind of the specialist who examined Robert that if things went on as they were a peptic ulcer would be the next logical development.

Although Robert's problems were perhaps slightly more serious than those of other children I've seen with stress problems his history is by no means unique. It is in fact extremely common these days for young children to be put under an unbearable amount of pressure to do well at school. The pressure is applied by both parents and schoolteachers and it covers sports and games as well as academic subjects.

It sometimes seems to me that hardly anyone plays games for fun any more, and there are today so many junior leagues and junior cups that even five and six-year-olds are encouraged to take their sports very seriously.

The same, of course, is quite true of adults who also seem to take their sports and games very seriously these days. A few years ago most of the men and women who played games no more than once or twice a week would really enjoy themselves, would describe themselves as merely social players and would relax on the squash court, the golf course or the football pitch. They would enjoy the camaraderie and the chance to do something different for a change as much as they would enjoy the competition. Today I find myself amazed whenever I go anywhere near a sports club of any kind. The people playing golf are worrying desperately about their handicaps and their latest scores. The squash players are to be found poring over instruction manuals and video recordings of their own games; and the football players are plunged into despair if they fail to pick up a trophy every season.

This desire to do well at everything, and to be seen to be doing well, is endemic in our modern society. The young executive who isn't ambitious is considered rather odd, and the man who enjoys his job, knows that he will be uncomfortable if he rises any higher in his company hierarchy, and refuses an unwanted promotion, will be considered irrational and very probably mentally ill rather than sensible and very sane.

The pressure to achieve begins to affect many of us at an early age, and it continues to affect us throughout our lives.

A question of belief: Annette Harkness

It may seem strange to suggest that religion can be a cause of stress – after all one of the traditional purposes of religion is to calm and soothe, to support and to provide guidance. But whatever the ideals and theoretical purposes of religion may be the simple truth is, I'm afraid, that religion is a common and very significant cause of stress in a great many people.

I could justify that claim in a number of different ways

but the simplest and perhaps the most obvious way is to describe a patient of mine who suffered greatly because of her religious beliefs.

Although she looked considerably older Mrs Annette Harkness was in her late twenties when I first met her. She had two small children and a husband to look after and all three seemed to lean on her a great deal. Before her marriage she had worked as a secretary in a building firm. She'd given up work when she was expecting her first child and although she had intended to go back to work later on she seemed to have few hopes of ever doing that when she joined my list of patients.

She'd given up her ambition to return to work because her second child had been born mentally handicapped and much of her life was spent in providing simple nursing care. She knew very well that her son, an unlucky victim of the whooping cough vaccine, was unlikely ever to manage to fend for himself.

All that may sound quite enough of a burden for one woman but Mrs Harkness had another huge problem to try and deal with. She was a Roman Catholic and her problem was that although she couldn't bear the idea of having any more children her Church taught that she would be quite wrong to use any form of contraception.

To begin with she trusted to luck and simply prayed every night not to get pregnant again. For a while it worked quite well, but one month she had a scare, was two weeks late with her period, and all her early terror of a third pregnancy returned.

That was more than enough for her. After that she refused to allow her husband to touch her and for three months she slept in the same bed as her mentally handicapped child. Each week when she saw the priest she asked him to allow her to use some form of contraception and each week he simply repeated what she already knew; that to use contraceptives would be to go against God and to incur the wrath of the Church.

Eventually the predictable happened and her husband had an affair with a divorced woman who worked as a barmaid in a local men's club. It wasn't so much a serious love affair as a simple case of lust, but it upset Mrs Harkness enough to convince her that she really ought to allow her husband back into her bed.

Whether the intervening period had made her more fertile or her God had acquired a more than mischievous sense of humour that single episode led to Mrs Harkness's third pregnancy.

To begin with Mrs Harkness was hysterical. She insisted that she couldn't possibly cope with a third child, that she couldn't go through another pregnancy. She sobbed and cried and pleaded for help.

Eventually, after she'd been interviewed several times by both an obstetrician and a psychiatrist she was offered an abortion. She accepted the offer immediately, had an abortion and returned home to the rage and disapproval of both her husband and her priest. They told her that she had sinned against God, that she was guilty of murder and that she would be damned for eternity.

Three weeks after the abortion she was admitted to hospital with a bleeding peptic ulcer, and four days later she died. The surgeon who had looked after her insisted that she had willed herself to death. He firmly believed that if she had had the slightest desire to live she would have survived.

I believe that Mrs Harkness could have survived if her only task had been to look after her family. She could have managed to look after her mentally handicapped child without too much difficulty. But the pressure of trying to reconcile her own needs, the needs of her husband and the teachings of the Church proved too much for her. For Mrs Harkness her faith was a burden she couldn't carry; it was directly responsible for a dilemma she couldn't solve, and by producing the pressure and stress which led to the development of her peptic ulcer, and the concomitant absence of any will to live, it led directly to her death.

Personal relationships: Alan Kent

When any close relationship between two people comes to an end the result can be catastrophic. The end of a love affair, the end of a marriage or the end of a friendship can all be extremely damaging in terms of the amount of stress they can produce. Obviously the closer the relationship the greater the damage that is done when the relationship comes to an end.

But it is not only when relationships end that stress is produced. In a marriage where the two partners are no longer in love with one another, or perhaps even more important when they no longer even like one another, the stresses and strains can be severe enough to produce any number of mental and physical problems.

Take Alan Kent, for example, who came to see me with clear and unmistakable signs of an early stomach ulcer, and told me how he and his wife had lived in a state of permanent feud for the better part of a year.

There hadn't been any particular reason for their falling out of love and into anger. In Mr Kent's own words 'it just seemed to happen over the years'. But whatever the cause may have been the effect was pretty daunting. Slowly over the months each partner had taken to nibbling at the other in the most hurtful and damaging way. Since they had not so long before been madly in love with one another they both knew where to bite in order to cause the maximum amount of pain.

Personal relationships are vital to us all. It is from our relationships with others that most of us obtain our strength.

But personal relationships that have gone sour for any reason can be a source of unending distress. And on the whole the closer the relationship is to start with the more acute the distress can be if it fails.

Pressure at work: John Elder

When we think of individuals who suffer from pressure at work we usually think of executives, company directors and others with too much responsibility. However, while it is of course true that people in positions of great power often do suffer from stress it is also true that those who work for them can often find themselves suffering from stress-induced diseases. As always it is not so much the type of stress or the nature of the work involved that is important as the attitude of the individual concerned and his or her capacity to cope with whatever levels of stress he may be expected to endure.

For five years Mr John Elder had driven a bus on a busy city route and for most of that time he had been accompanied on his journeys by a conductor. Mr Elder had been responsible for driving the bus and for making sure that the company's schedules were kept, and the conductor's job was to ensure that each passenger paid the correct fare.

Mr Elder's problems arose when the company decided to save some money by introducing a fleet of pay-as-you-enter buses. For Mr Elder this was a very significant change. Instead of simply having to cope with driving his bus through the busy city traffic, he now also had the responsibility of taking money from would-be passengers and providing them with tickets.

He found that this was by no means as easy a task as it sounds. One major problem was that many of the people who got onto the bus didn't have the correct change and would argue angrily when he pointed to the notice informing would-be passengers that only people carrying the right coins would be allowed to ride on the bus. On several occasions Mr Elder found himself being threatened and eventually he gave up arguing with passengers and simply provided the change if it was required. This in turn made him unpopular with the other drivers who were sticking rigidly to the regulations.

After two weeks of this Mr Elder came to my surgery complaining of stomach pains. He was obviously very distressed and, in addition to giving him a supply of antacid tablets designed to relieve the immediate discomfort, I provided him with a sick note for work, suggesting that he should take at least a fortnight off duty.

When, two weeks later, Mr Elder returned to the surgery he seemed a different man. He looked very much better and said he felt much improved. He was eager to get back to work, so I provided him with a certificate stating that he was fit to start driving his bus again.

That, unfortunately, was when his problems returned. Within three days of starting back to work and finding himself besieged by angry passengers Mr Elder was back in my consulting room pleading for more antacid tablets and another sick note.

I think it is entirely reasonable to assume that the stress of driving a pay-as-you-enter bus had caused Mr Elder's stomach symptoms. The symptoms had, after all, developed within a few days of his starting the new job, they had disappeared when he'd stayed away from work, and they had returned when he'd gone back to work.

The Micawber principle: Peter Nixon

There are relatively few people in our society who are in genuine danger of starving to death because they cannot afford to buy enough food to eat, or of freezing to death because they don't have any shelter or enough money to pay for basic heating.

But there are a great many people who are quite genu-
inely worried and distressed because they have money problems with which they cannot cope. Some of those individuals
suffer because for one reason or another their income is totally
inadequate to enable them to cope with ordinary living expenses.
And some suffer because through no real fault of their own
they are hit by unexpected demands and expenses.

More numerous than individuals in these categories, however, and perhaps even more likely to suffer from stress-induced
illnesses as a result of their financial problems, are those people
who have an adequate income but who for one reason or another struggle to live beyond their means.

Encouraged to spend and buy items that they may not
need or even want, many people who could theoretically live
comfortably on their earnings, push themselves into debt. Se-
duced by the banks who regularly use advertising to encourage
people to borrow money to pay for luxury items, these individuals push themselves further and further into debt and deeper
into trouble. Encouraged by easy-term higher purchase arrangements they buy equipment they don't need with money they
haven't got.

If one partner in a marriage wants to spend and the other
wants to save the agonies and pressure can mount even more
rapidly. The partner who wants to spend will accuse the partner who wants to save of being mean and miserly while the one
who wants to save will accuse the other of being profligate and
careless. Whatever the end result may be the consequences in
terms of the partnership can be devastating.

Peter Nixon and his wife Petronella had been married for
just three years when their marriage fell apart. Peter had a
modest position with a large national company. Petronella was
far more ambitious than her husband. She insisted that they
live in a house they could not afford and drive a car which was
financially beyond them. She acquired friends who were much

wealthier and her financial demands put an unbearable strain on her husband and her marriage. Eventually Peter fell ill with stomach and bowel problems.

Sexual problems: Dawn Glidway

Few causes of stress are as invasive or as ubiquitous as sex. It gets everywhere, affects everything, and has an overall influence far greater than any of us might imagine were we to try and assess its status and significance in our lives.

Sex, is for example, one of the main weapons used by advertising copywriters, packagers and marketing men. It is more difficult to think of an item that isn't sold with the aid of sex than to think of one that is.

Even when advertising doesn't obviously and directly use sex to sell us a product, sex is usually in there somewhere. Advertisements for soaps and mouthwashes, for example, will usually imply that if you don't use the right product you'll be unlikely to attract the partner of your choice.

All this advertising pressure produces results, of course. But it doesn't just sell the products that it is designed to sell. It also encourages a wide range of suspicions, fears and fantasies about sex.

It is, for example, not at all unknown for individuals to consider themselves to be in some way exceptional or odd because they do not spend their days thinking about sex and their nights practising what they have been thinking. And with the pressure from the advertisers, allied with the pressure from all those sex marketeers who have a commercial interest in selling us sexual delights of every possible kind, it is hardly surprising that there are today a great many men and women who worry because their own sexual activities are seemingly unexceptional both in quality and quantity.

Indeed, it is, in my experience, far more common for individuals to be worried about the fact that they don't seem to be as interested in sex, or as determined to experiment in sexual matters as they think they ought to be, than it is for people to be worried by a genuine equipment failure of some kind. The majority of people think they have a sexual problem only because their own attitudes, ambitions and yearnings don't match up to the attitudes, ambitions and yearnings that they think they ought to experience. The advertisers and the marketeers have between them created a new type of pressure and have produced a whole range of sexual problems.

Dawn Glidway was happy with her husband, her marriage and her sex life until she started reading about multiple orgasms in a monthly magazine. From that moment on poor Dennis Glidway's life became quite miserable. His wife's new expectations were hardly ever fulfilled and since there was no one else available he got the blame and developed a persistent stomach problem.

Women's liberation: Fiona Willings

The other sexual problem which can't be ignored is nothing to do with raw sexuality but is instead a product of the fairly modern liberation movement.

During recent years a growing number of women have begun to demand and expect to be treated as individuals with rights and responsibilities of their own rather than to be treated simply as companions, wives or mistresses. Quite justifiably those women who have taken an active part in the emancipation movement have campaigned for equality in all areas of living.

Unfortunately, the problems which have arisen from this type of campaign have affected both women and men and have produced many heartaches and much concern.

Women who might a few years ago have been relatively content simply to regard themselves as mothers and housewives now feel that if they are to live their lives to the full they should enjoy a career outside the home. This has nothing to do with the need for extra money (although that is obviously another cause of stress) but is simply a question of achieving status as an individual human being.

The problem is, of course, that many of the women who have recently tried to combine looking after a home with resuming a career have found themselves torn between their two sets of duties. On the one hand they have been anxious to carve out for themselves some sort of personal career. On the other hand they have found themselves struggling to satisfy the demands of their husbands and families. The amount of guilt and the amount of stress produced by that guilt has been enormous. When Fiona Willings had a baby she really wanted to stay at home and be a mother and a wife. But her mother and her sister were both committed members of the Women's Liberation Movement and Fiona felt that she had no choice but to resume her career within days of her baby's birth. The result was that Fiona, desperately trying to be all things to all men (and women), was constantly filled with guilt and troubled by persistent indigestion.

At the same time a large number of men have found themselves facing almost identical problems. They have been conscious of the fact that they have a duty to allow their wives to run their own lives and yet they have still felt a duty to provide and to be protective. All that has produced some very considerable psychological problems.

The modern environment: Julie Young

Our ancestors had to live in surroundings far less well organised than our own and it does seem somehow to be rather churlish if we complain about the stressful nature of the environment in which we live. It looks as though we are just being difficult to please if we complain that life in a big, modern city with its piped water, electricity and music is as stressful as life was in, say, a small medieval town with primitive sewage facilities, unmade roads and no public facilities to speak of.

And yet I do believe that life in a modern, big city is probably more stressful than life in those relatively primitive surroundings.

There are several reasons for this, of course. Our own demands and expectations, and those of the people around us, are very different to the demands of our ancestors. The pace of modern living is much faster. And the number of problems and pressures is considerably greater today than it was a few centuries ago.

Julie Young married at the age of seventeen and very rapidly had two children. By the time she'd reached the grand old age of twenty she was an experienced, harassed and slightly world-weary mother. She lived in a small apartment on the nineteenth storey of a block of flats, and despite having to put up with all the usual problems associated with bringing up children while living so far above the ground she seemed to sail through life without too many problems.

When I first heard her complain of what sounded like fairly ordinary indigestion I initially blamed her diet which seemed to consist largely of a very unhealthy mixture of cigarettes, cheap wine and chips. She seemed a calm, phlegmatic young woman and I had no reason to suspect that she was suffering from stress. I advised her to try and consume a slightly more nutritious diet and I prescribed an ordinary antacid for her to try.

That didn't really help very much, however, and a month later she was still suffering from exactly the same symptoms. Neither my dietary advice nor my prescription had helped.

We sat down together for half an hour and tried to work out precisely what might be causing her symptoms. And eventually she confessed that what was really worrying her was a story she'd read in a national newspaper. The story had described how a small boy had fallen from a balcony of a flat on the fourteenth storey of a block in the north of England. Since reading the story she'd been absolutely terrified of leaving her children alone for more than a minute or two and she'd become absolutely obsessed about locking the door to their tiny balcony.

Her new habits had simply made things worse. Her husband was getting fed up with having to spend ages hunting for the key every time he wanted to go out onto the balcony to look at his tomato plants and Mrs Young herself was finding her obsession an enormous burden. On several occasions she'd found herself making her way back up to the nineteenth floor to check on the balcony door even though the children hadn't been left in the apartment.

It was only when she revealed her fears to me that I realised that her indigestion symptoms had very probably been produced by her stress and anxiety about the children. When I managed to help arrange for her balcony to be fitted with childproof railings the indigestion symptoms disappeared entirely.

Mrs Young illustrates very clearly the point I want to make. For even though I feel confident that her indigestion symptoms were produced by stress there is no way in which I can prove the connection conclusively. There is strong circumstantial evidence in that the pains were present when she was worrying and they disappeared when she stopped worrying. But that doesn't provide solid scientific proof that stress caused damage to her stomach.

***

The biggest cause of stress in a modern city comes from the fact that so many of the things which cause pressure are out of our own control. If you live in a town where the roads are badly made, and you know that they are badly made, then you get accustomed to getting your feet muddy and you either get used to that or you wear something to protect your feet. Paved roads don't exist so there is no solution to the problem as far as you're concerned. You must do the best that you can to make life bearable and to minimise the amount of stress. Similarly if there isn't any public sewage system then you must make your own arrangements. You dig your own hole and when it is full you dig another. The problem is soluble and you are not reliant on anyone else. When you need heat you chop up wood, and when you run out of wood you chop up more. You know precisely what you have to do to maintain your living standard and your reliance on others is very limited.

In a modern city, however, things are very different. The problems and the pressures are neither easily solved nor are they easily dismissed. Many continue to irritate and annoy from day to day. Our reliance on one another, for example, means that when something goes wrong with the plumbing, or when there is an electricity strike, or when the rubbish is not collected, problems sprout alarmingly. The absence of electricity can mean an absence of heat and light, and since we have all grown up to be dependent upon piped facilities such as water, gas and electricity our capacity to cope when the supply is withdrawn is severely limited. With things out of our control the problems produce stresses of almost incalculable magnitude.

In the days when people who wanted to travel from one place to another had either to walk or to ride on horseback, there were enormous problems in travelling long distances. But those problems were easily defined and everyone knew what they were. Expectations were very limited and it was up to the individual himself to make his own arrangements to travel.

Today most of us travel more in a week than our ancestors would have travelled in a year. We expect to be able to travel long distances in fairly short periods of time. We become very stressed if for any reason there is a breakdown in the transport system or a traffic queue causes a hold-up. Our personal expectations are high but our capacity to do anything to ensure that our expectations are met is strictly limited. If the trains aren't running, or the buses aren't available, or there is a strike at the airport, then there are no simple solutions to the many problems which result. If you're stuck in a traffic jam twenty miles away from the office then there is nothing much you can do about it. If you live on the tenth floor of a block of flats and you have a baby in a pushchair, or you suffer from arthritis, then you are entirely dependent on the lift working. If the lift doesn't work then you're marooned ten storeys up and there is absolutely nothing you can do about it yourself, except walk up and down the stairs.

New machinery produces noise and pollutions of many other kinds. There are increased risks of accidents occurring in heavily populated city areas where motor cars run in great profusion. The more sophisticated and complicated our environment becomes the more numerous are the problems which develop.

Progress: A constant source of anxiety

Every development which adds to the complexity of modern life (and which admittedly may be designed to improve the quality of life) makes each one of us more and more dependent upon our neighbours and upon the others living in and working in the same local and national community. Ironically and tragically the machines and equipment designed to assist those who work on our behalf are now often so complicated and so sophisticated that it is the machines which are the principals in the provision of services and the human beings who are there to assist. This reversal of the traditional relationship between men and machines means that individuals are often so bored by the work that they do, and so deprived of any real sense of satisfaction, that they are likely to strike (and thereby create additional problems for thousands of fellow citizens) in order to establish their own identity. The better a city's facilities become the more likely it is that there will be problems, and the more certain it is that those problems will adversely affect large numbers of people.

All of this may be of little comfort next time you are stuck in a bus queue or stranded ten floors up without a lift or any electricity but it does, I hope, illustrate just why living in a modern, twentieth-century city can be far more stressful than living in a primitive community. Problems you can solve yourself produce relatively little stress because there is only limited opportunity for frustration to develop. Problems that you cannot solve without the cooperation of others become immensely frustrating, and therefore immensely stressful, if the cooperation of those others is withheld for any reason.

The changing world

While writing this book I took time out one day to clear out some of the shelves in my study. I'm an inveterate book collector and from time to time the piles of books on the floor become too numerous and too high for me to move around without causing a series of minor avalanches. So I set about sorting through some of the books on the shelves in order to select volumes which could safely be moved into the cupboard under the stairs.

What amazed me most on my purge along the shelves was the discovery that the majority of the textbooks that I had used when I was a medical student in the late 1960s were quite out of date. My guide to diseases of the stomach gave much space to the possible causes of duodenal ulcers but never mentioned stress or worry. My surgery textbook had been published when transplantation was a horticultural term. My psychiatry textbooks recommended brain surgery for disorders such as peptic ulceration and anxiety. My pharmacology textbook contained no mention of many, popular, modern drugs. The textbook which I used as a general introduction to medicine had nothing in it about endoscopy – now a routine investigative procedure. Just about the only textbooks which were still of any value were the anatomy texts. Things have changed so rapidly in the world of medicine that books which were considered accurate and up-to-date are now just so much worthless paper of interest only to historians. Indeed, in some instances they are dangerous rather than useful.

If you stop and think about it for a minute or two you will quickly realise that it is not just in medicine or education that changes are taking place at a tremendous rate. In just about all aspects of life change is such a normal and readily accepted part of living that children who have grown up in the last few decades automatically assume that the things that they learn today will be just so much history by tomorrow. They expect and are accustomed to a world in which dolls, toys, clothes, records, books and television personalities move in and out of fashion with no more chance of permanence than snowflakes.

All this transience, novelty and diversity has meant that the speed of living has changed and many people have found themselves in an almost permanent state of shock as they struggle to cope with the fact that aspects of life which they had formerly regarded as settled have now suddenly become as unstable and unpredictable as the world of *haute couture*. Inflation, economic revolutions, changes in measurement standards, the development and wider availability of computers – all these things have meant that life has become unbearably fast for some people. Some even find the fact that we live in a world dominated by disposables difficult to accept, and I have met many individuals who have been deeply worried by the thought of people buying and then throwing away such items as pens, razors, lighters and torches.

It is not possible to halt change, of course, even though not all change can be regarded as progress. But by being aware of the fact that we live in an ever-changing society, by determining to maintain some certainty and structure in our own lives and by building up our own capacity for stress control we can all improve our chances of coping and surviving.

Boredom

Whenever I talk about stress and its causes in public I always find there is a general assumption that people only really suffer from stress-induced illnesses when something is actually happening to them. Over the years most people seem to have come to regard stress as something only endured by harassed businessmen, overworked schoolteachers, housewives under pressure and others whose lives are conducted at a great pace.

Mention the word stress to most people and, as I've pointed out earlier in this book, they will think of businessmen holding meetings in hotel corridors and nursing headaches, high blood pressure and stomach ulcers. Stress is something most of us associate with activity and according to our own personal experiences we may, when we think of stress, think of screaming children, bundles of wet nappies and broken-down washing machines or piles of untyped letters, broken-down printers and angry employers.

All that is true, of course. It is a fact that an individual who is under excessive pressure will quite probably suffer from one or more stress-induced diseases. The businessman may have high blood pressure, the young mother under pressure may develop a migraine headache and the secretary who can no longer cope with her workload may end up with colitis.

But just as too much activity can cause stress so can too little activity. And just as too much pressure can produce physical and mental damage so a lack of pressure can, paradoxi-cally, produce exactly the same effect.

Having studied individuals under stress for many years now I'm convinced that boredom is indeed just about the single largest cause of stress in our modern society.

Consider, for example, all those individuals who find their daily work less than satisfying. How many people can possibly say that they enjoy every aspect of their work? Not many, I suspect. Just consider the workforce in the average car compo-nent factory. On the shop floor the employee probably works alongside sophisticated pieces of machinery which do most of the difficult work and need to be fed with raw materials, given regular supplies of oil and maintained in good working order. Conveyor belts probably carry bits and pieces of partly com-pleted machinery from one part of the factory floor to another. The whole process of manufacture will be geared to the needs and capabilities of the machines rather than of the men oper-ating them.

Men who might have once been regarded as skilled crafts-men are today employed as simple machine minders, babysitting several thousand pounds' worth of highly complicated engi-neering and helping to produce small pieces of metal in which they can take no personal pride.

In the offices the white-collar workers are similarly sub-servient to machines. Instead of machines which make indi-vidual items there are computers and word processors which need to be fed with information and instructions. In the office, as on the factory floor, the machine is in charge.

Understandably anxious to compete with the production schedules met by their competitors, manufacturers install more and more machinery each year. And as those machines take over the most interesting and rewarding jobs, so the people employed in those factories are more likely to become bored by their work. Machines were once used to assist men; today men are employed to assist and look after the machines. It is hardly surprising that in well-organised factories where craftsmen are no longer employed, and where job satisfaction is limited to the size of the pay packet, strikes are common. Employees, whether they are working on the factory floor or in the offices, are frustrated by their lack of responsibility and the absence of any real sense of satisfaction in the work they do. The only chance they have to obtain some sense of satisfaction is by using their very presence as a weapon and by continually demanding shorter working hours and larger pay packets. The lack of identity and boredom which are common problems in such factories can only be relieved by striking.

Those who work at home are not exempt from boredom.

Housewives probably make up the largest single group of individuals who are likely to be affected by boredom.

I realise that many thousands of women reading that sentence will probably react indignantly and quickly point out that they don't have time to be bored. They are far too busy making the beds, picking up bits of dirty laundry, preparing meals, washing up, cleaning the house, making sure that everyone has clean handkerchiefs and fresh socks, polishing windows, and doing the thousand and one other chores which make up part of the housewife's daily duties.

Now, I am very happy to agree that all those activities will probably keep the average housewife busy. She'll undoubtedly be kept rushing round the house from the moment she gets up in the morning to the time when she flops down into an easy chair late at night. But I wonder how many of those scurrying housewives would argue that they find their household chores satisfying, or would claim that they actually enjoy washing up and polishing the floors? I wonder how many would claim that they get real satisfaction from throwing armfuls of dirty washing into the washing machine and then ironing what doesn't get chewed up by the tumble dryer?

And how many would agree with me that, however worthwhile, most of these duties are dull, undemanding and boring?

***

Stress does not disappear when we retire. And nor does boredom.

I regularly read about trade union officials claiming that their members should be allowed to retire early, and today it is by no means uncommon for men and women who are in their fifties to strap on their gold watches and hang up their working clothes. I always wonder if those trade union officials realise exactly what they are doing for their members when they campaign so ferociously for early retirement.

For although many individuals gain little enough satisfaction from their daily work they gain even less from their lives once they have put on their carpet slippers and left work for good. The man or woman who has retired will often consider him or herself to be in some way unwanted. There is no status in retirement and too few individuals have the capacity to carve out a meaningful life for themselves once they have left work for good.

Walk into an old people's home almost anywhere and look around you. You'll see row after row of sad, bored faces belonging to sad, bored old people who have nothing more exciting to do than complain about the quality of the gravy, moan about the unknown thief who took their favourite newspaper and mutter about the woman across the room who won't stop taking out her false teeth and cleaning them on her jumper. Boredom in old people's homes is the biggest threat to health and sanity, and yet it is something that men and women who keep working into their seventies, eighties and even nineties hardly ever know.

***

Those examples aren't intended to be exhaustive by any means. Boredom is a problem that affects us all from time to time. Those three groups of people just happen to be the largest groups of individuals who are particularly likely to suffer stress as a result of their boredom.

The housewife who gets little satisfaction from her housework, who spends her time operating machines she doesn't understand, opening packets of instant food she doesn't like, and who lives on a housing estate where each family lives in an isolated block and plaster cell will become disillusioned, depressed and bored.

The factory worker or office clerk who spends his or her time serving the needs of complex machines and who gets about as much job satisfaction as the machine itself will become disillusioned, depressed and bored.

And the man or woman who has taken early retirement and who spends his or her time waiting for the next television programme to start, and then complaining about it, will also become disillusioned, depressed and bored.

For all these individuals it is the absence of pressure that has done the damage. Frustrated by the absence of any real test or trial for their talents they will become increasingly anxious as their awareness of the futility of their lives is matched by the feeling that somehow they are being cheated of success and satisfaction.

Their boredom can lead to any one of the many disorders associated with stress.

The four cornerstones: Kenny Orville

I have often argued that our lives are built upon four cornerstones (home, work, friendship and hobbies) and that when more than one of those cornerstones is affected at the same time the chances of a patient suffering serious stress-related problems is unusually high.

One patient of mine exhibited only too well the sort of

problems which can arise when two or more of the four corner-stones are disturbed at the same time.

Kenny Orville had been married for seven years when I first saw him and had worked for a year longer than that in the same office of a large travel agency.

His marriage had slowly been crumbling for nearly half its length, and it finally fell apart as a result of a row about whether or not the Orvilles should have their annual summer holiday in France or Germany. It had been an unhappy marriage for some time and I don't think either partner was entirely sad to see the relationship finally and formally broken.

In some ways Kenny was actually relieved that he no longer had to go on pretending to love the woman with whom he lived and I suspect that the break up of his marriage would, had it been the only major event in his life at the time, have been of remarkably little consequence to him.

However, two days after his marriage had finally fallen apart Kenny fulfilled the ambition of his working life and told his employer exactly what he thought of him. He also told him precisely what he could do with his job. This quite naturally meant that Kenny was now not only separated but also unemployed, and since most of his friends worked at the travel agency it also meant that he was separated from them as well.

When he came to see me a week after all this had happened Kenny Orville was suffering from quite acute pains in his upper abdomen. He was feeling nauseated most of the time and his appetite had more or less disappeared although he was swallowing biscuits by the handful and glasses of milk by the dozen in a vain attempt to keep the pain in his stomach under control. When I talked to him he admitted that he had suffered from various pains in his upper abdomen for the best part of nine months but he insisted that none of the pains had been anywhere near as bad as the one that he had developed in the last few days.

A few hours later Kenny's peptic ulcer perforated and he needed an operation in order to repair the damage that had been done. Now it is, of course, quite impossible to prove that Kenny's sudden deterioration was directly connected to the loss of three of his life's cornerstones, but in my view it was no coincidence that his stomach problem deteriorated when it did. Kenny had made the potentially fatal mistake of making dramatic changes in several important parts of his life at the same time. The resultant stress had been too much for his stomach to bear and Kenny had suffered accordingly.

Lifestyle changes: Peter Roberts

Peter Roberts was another patient of mine whose stomach problems became much worse when he made dramatic changes in his lifestyle. Peter worked as a sales representative for a food manufacturer and he was, I understand, extremely good at his job. He was certainly good enough to impress his superiors in the firm for they promoted him to a job as sales manager in another part of the country. Now, although it may be rather difficult for people who are unemployed to accept, getting promoted can be an extremely stressful business. And Peter Roberts tackled his promotion in a way almost designed to ensure that all his family felt the stresses as acutely as possible.

Two days after he had been informed of his promotion Peter took his wife and their two nine-year-old twin daughters down to the area where he was going to be sales manager and started house hunting. The company for which he worked was a large international concern which didn't like its employees to hang around, so Peter had something like two weeks in which to prepare and plan his move.

Now as anyone who has ever moved house will confirm there are a good many problems to be overcome. There are the legal and contractual problems associated with selling one home and buying another. There are the problems of buying carpets and curtains, arranging for furniture removers to call, informing the telephone company, the gas people and the electricity suppliers, and of course, finding a new school. To try and manage all this in a single two-week period is expecting a good deal of everyone concerned. To try and manage it all in a single two-week period while you're tying up the loose ends from one job and preparing to start unravelling the loose ends from another job, as Peter Roberts was, is asking for trouble.

And Peter Roberts found his trouble. He ended up spending the day he should have been moving house in the local hospitals being investigated for chest pains. It was thought at first that the pains were due to heart trouble. It was only later that it became clear that what he had really been suffering from was severe indigestion caused by stress.

He would, perhaps, have been wiser to have moved into a hotel in the area where he was going to work and to have settled into his new job first before trying to move house and home. The stress of commuting and being away from his family during the week would almost certainly have been less than the stress of trying to cope with a major upheaval involving all four cornerstones at once.

An inability to say 'no': June Harper

June Harper was a foreman in a local car component factory and she hated her job. She had accepted the post only because no one else really wanted it and she had not had the temerity to refuse when the firm's works manager had offered it to her. She found the job distasteful because she was now isolated from her former friends yet still not part of the management hierarchy. She felt that she was in a limbo in between the shop floor and the top level management group.

In addition to her position as a works foreman Mrs Harper

was also a member of an enormous range of committees. She was secretary of her local Women's Institute Group, treasurer of the Parent-Teacher's Association, and on half-a-dozen other assorted committees. Whenever there was a local flag-day to organise on behalf of some charity or other she would find herself standing around with a can and a tray of flowers. Most of her weekday evenings were spent sitting either in draughty church halls listening to boring speeches or in a spare bedroom at home going through sheaves of paperwork. She didn't like the committee work or the paperwork, and she found herself getting more and more stressed by the fact that so many people seemed determined to impose on her goodwill.

I asked her why she had allowed herself to get involved in so many activities that she didn't enjoy and she confessed that the reason was really quite simple. She just couldn't say 'no'.

'I always feel so guilty,' she confessed. 'People ask me to do things and although I don't really want to do them at all I say 'yes' because I don't want to be rude or offensive'.

There are lots of people like Mrs Harper, and unfortunately there are also lots of people who are prepared to take advantage of those who find it too difficult to say 'no'.

In general, I think that it is fair to say that the people who suffer most from this inability to avoid getting committed to projects in which they themselves have no real interest are those individuals who are over blessed with such good qualities as generosity, kindness and compassion.

There is no simple answer to this particular type of problem, of course, for if you are the sort of person who finds it difficult to say 'no' then you really aren't ever going to find it easy to turn down requests for help.

Still, you should try. Practise saying 'Thank you, but no'. And you might find it easier if you remember that the people who keep asking for your help are simply taking advantage of your generous nature.

Be careful how you relax: Roderick Burns

Roderick Burns worked as a factory manager and he had a proven peptic ulcer about two years ago. He took drugs for a few months but eventually needed an operation. After the operation he swore that he would relax a little more and take life a little more gently.

To help him do just that he bought a small cottage in the country where he assured me he would be able to get away from all his problems. And he was quite right in that he certainly did get away from his problems at work. But all he did was exchange his worries about the factory for worries about his cottage. The drainpipes got blocked regularly with leaves from trees. The roof leaked on two occasions. Part of the chimney stack fell in. There was dry rot in the kitchen. The problems just went on and on and Mr Burns found himself worrying just as much about his cottage as he was worrying about his job.

It shouldn't have been a big surprise to anyone when he acquired a second peptic ulcer.

He had failed to realise that there is very little point in exchanging one set of stresses for another set of stresses. What Roderick needed was not another bunch of problems to worry about but a few days complete break every now and again. He would have benefited much more if he had chosen to spend his holidays in hotels or boarding houses where he could have allowed himself to relax properly, and where he could have forgotten his worries and problems completely.

Indeed, he would probably have had a much more beneficial break if he had stayed at home, switched off the telephone, locked the front door and settled down with a pile of good books and magazines to read.

(Incidentally, before leaving the subject of 'escape' I must mention the fact that many very busy people have learned to escape from their day-to-day worries for a few minutes at a time by using children's games. Executive toys are something of a joke to some people but they do help a great deal by enabling the executive to regress to his childhood in a moment of crisis. The fact that the toys are well-made and expensive means that he can do this without losing any status.

I firmly believe that children's toys such as puzzles and other games are an excellent way to switch off from problems that are causing tremendous stress. And by offering a minor challenge on a completely different level they allow the individual concerned to regain his strength and to return to the original, main problem with renewed vigour and recharged batteries. My study is littered with games and puzzles of all kinds.)

Stored up emotions: George Young

Forty years ago George Young had a small market stall on which he sold all sorts of miscellaneous items. Through hard work and a considerable amount of business acumen he built up his business from that single market stall until it consisted of a chain of retail shops selling groceries.

He was justifiably proud of that chain of stores and it was, I know, with some regret that he eventually accepted a bid from a huge international company which wanted to add his chain to their own collection of stores. I don't think he would have accepted the offer at all if he had had any children but since he had no heir he was, I think, well aware that the shops eventually had to be managed by someone else.

While negotiating the sale of his shops George had successfully managed to persuade the directors of the major company to allow him to continue to run his own business. He wanted to run things in much the same sort of way that he had always done and the international company was keen enough to buy his stores to agree to his request.

When the takeover finally took place, therefore, George

was really not too upset. He still imagined that he would have very much the same sort of control over the day-to-day running of his shops as he had had before and he still thought of them as 'his' shops.

But, of course, that's not the way big business is run; within two days of the takeover being completed the big international company had sent round a team of men to take down the signs over George's shops and replace them with their own signs. The day after that they sent round a psychologist to vet all the staff and the day after that they began to organise an army of shopfitters whose task it was to strip all the shops to the walls and refurnish them entirely.

George was horrified and when he heard what was going on he immediately telephoned the chairman of the international company that had bought his shops. That was when he discovered how different things were really going to be now that the trading courtship was over. The chairman, who prior to the takeover had happily taken all his calls, laughed at all his jokes and been enthusiastic about every one of George's pet projects, was suddenly unavailable. George found himself talking to an assistant; a young man with a haughty manner, a condescending voice and a total disregard for George's own ambitions, hopes and aspirations.

That was just the beginning. Things slowly got worse during the days and weeks that followed. George found that although he had expected to be allowed to have some day-to-day control over his shops he was, in practice, given virtually no control at all. Buying was all done from a central department. Advertising was organised by an agency. Staff recruitment was managed by a 'human resources department'. And George found himself sitting in his own expensively furnished office playing with the paperclips.

To begin with he managed to disguise from his colleagues and friends the extent of his disappointment. At the golf club he remained his usual quietly humorous self. At home he managed to exhibit tremendous self-control. There were no signs anywhere of his sadness and sorrow and none of those close to him had any idea that George was suffering.

He came to me for help because although he was managing to cope well with his problems George suddenly found himself experiencing extraordinary feelings of violence. He had never hit anyone in anger in his life and yet suddenly he found himself worrying that he might suddenly kill someone.

The fears were so real that he found himself in a cold sweat every time he passed the tool bench in the garage or saw a knife in the kitchen. And what made these strange feelings so remarkable and so terrifying as far as George was concerned was the fact that the person he felt that he wanted to kill was his wife.

'Why do I want to kill her?' George wanted to know. 'Why don't I want to kill the chairman of that damned company. Or his wretched young assistant?'

I explained to him that he was displacing the anger and frustration that he felt, and that it was because he had made such an effort to disguise his feelings towards his new employer that George found himself unable even to enjoy the idea of destroying him in a fantasy. George's determination to disguise his personal feelings had left him twisted and distorted inside and he was subconsciously attempting to redirect some of that anger. His wife just happened to be the closest person to him and therefore the most likely target for his displaced aggression.

I've related that story because I think it illustrates very well why we should always endeavour to let our feelings out rather than bottle them up inside us. When I saw George he was beginning to feel guilty because of his apparently inexplicable feelings towards his wife. Before long he would have probably begun to resent the fact that she was unwittingly making him feel guilty. And so it would have gone on.

It could have all been avoided if only George had allowed

himself to get rid of his feelings of anger and annoyance rather more naturally. If he'd screamed and shouted at the chairman's assistant, or if he'd thrown a tantrum, he would have lost a little dignity but he might have felt very much better afterwards. And, most important of all, he would have got some aggression out of his system.

But for many people like George, of course, it isn't that easy to allow emotional feelings to show. After all we are often taught as children that we should always try to hide our emotions. We are taught that it is wrong to allow others to see us getting angry. Children, and boys in particular, are taught that it is wrong to cry in public. And there seems to be a very well-established tradition that it is much better to bottle up fears, anxieties and anger, and suffer in silence, rather than to let ourselves go and let others see just how we feel.

I firmly believe that bottling up emotions like this produces two types of damage. To begin with I think that it is partly because of the fact that we all try to hide our emotions from one another that there is so much violence in our society. One particular type of violence that often occurs more or less directly as a result of emotions being bottled up is baby battering. The young mother who is alone and worried and not really capable of coping with her child will often store up so much anger against the world in general that eventually she just takes it all out on her baby.

And I also believe that bottled up emotions can cause internal damage too, producing all the standard stress-induced diseases such as headaches, asthma and peptic ulcers. If you are an ulcer victim or an indigestion sufferer and you have a tendency to bottle up your feelings and refrain from letting other people know how you feel then I think that there is a very good chance that the two things are related. Your stored emotional feelings are very probably responsible for your stomach symptoms.

PART THREE

PROBLEMS AFFECTING THE STOMACH AND UPPER INTESTINAL TRACT

'Indigestion, n. A disease which the patient and his friends frequently mistake for deep religious conviction and concern for the salvation of mankind. As the simple Red Man of the western wild put it, with, it must be confessed, a certain force: 'Plenty well, no pray; big bellyache, heap God.'
AMBROSE BIERCE (1842–?1914), IN *THE DEVIL'S DICTIONARY*

Duodenal ulcer

The most important symptom of a duodenal ulcer is usually pain, and indeed this is often the only symptom that occurs. The pain is usually localized in the epigastrium, a central point about half way between the chin and the umbilicus (navel) and, unlike gastric ulcers, eating usually helps relieve the pain. People who have duodenal ulcers will often wake up at night and sneak downstairs to get a glass of milk and a biscuit.

The other characteristic factor of the pain that people get with duodenal ulceration is that it tends to disappear for weeks or even months at a time for no very apparent reason. Suddenly, just when you thought it had gone away for ever back it comes with a bang!

Gastric ulcer

The stomach lining or mucosa can be damaged by a number of different factors – tobacco, alcohol and fats, for example. This explains why individuals who have gastric ulcers will usually get better quicker if they cut out cigarettes and alcohol and if they steer away from fatty foods as much as possible.

Gastric ulcer pain is usually localized to the epigastrium and eating usually makes it worse. Unlike duodenal ulcer pain, gastric ulcer pain doesn't usually go away once it has started.

Gastritis

Gastritis is an inflammation of the stomach that can be produced by alcohol, by the consumption of a foodstuff to which you are allergic, by a virus infection or by any one of a number of other mechanisms which are not yet properly understood. There are some specific changes in the stomach mucosa when gastritis is present, but in practice it is virtually impossible to differentiate clinically between dyspepsia, gastritis and peptic ulcers without undergoing specific investigations such as a barium meal examination or an endoscopy (see page 75).

Heartburn

Under normal circumstances the acid mixture that helps to digest food within the stomach is kept away from the oesophagus by a sphincter which allows food to travel down into the stomach but doesn't allow food and acid to travel upwards into the gullet. The acid in the stomach is strong enough to dissolve steak (or burn holes in your carpet) and the oesophagus simply isn't made to cope with it. The sphincter is important. If the sphincter which usually divides the oesophagus from the stomach in this way doesn't do its job properly acid can sometimes splash upwards and irritate the oesophageal mucosa. The technical term for this is gastro-oesophageal reflux and the word 'heartburn' is very descriptive. The burning sensation rises up from the stomach and radiates to the upper chest – sometimes producing such a vicious pain that it can be confused with a heart attack.

Even when the sphincter is in good working condition acid can irritate the oesophagus when you lie down or bend over. Naturally enough, therefore, individuals who have a weak sphincter at that point will find that they suffer far more when they are lying flat or bending over than they do when they are standing up straight. Being overweight can increase the risk of heartburn. As can eating a diet which contains too much fat. And there are many individuals who suffer from this symptom purely as a result of stress.

As many as one in ten adults has reflux symptoms on a daily basis. Nearly half get symptoms at least once a month. Pregnant women are particularly at risk and around three quarters of pregnant women suffer from heartburn at some point in their pregnancy. Heartburn is a widespread and major problem. If it persists heartburn can be associated with ear pain, asthma, sinusitis and chronic laryngitis.

Indigestion (dyspepsia)

This isn't a word that doctors use a great deal when describing stomach problems because it is a particularly vague sort of word which doesn't really mean anything definite. In literal terms the word indigestion simply means that there has been a failure of digestion and so it can theoretically refer to problems in the intestinal tract further on than the stomach.

In practice, the word is used to describe the sort of symptoms which occur when a meal is eaten too quickly or after a particularly spicy or fatty meal.

Sufferers usually complain of some pain in the centre of

the chest and they may also feel slightly bloated. It's common for indigestion sufferers to complain of excessive wind and nausea. Occasionally an indigestion sufferer will actually vomit. Very few people who have indigestion will be interested in food for the pain tends to be accompanied by a full feeling and a loss of appetite.

Indigestion can be caused by smoking too much, by drinking too much alcohol or by taking too much tea or coffee. Other drugs, such as aspirin, can also cause indigestion.

However, although these specific causes are significant many of the individuals who suffer from indigestion do so directly as a result of stress.

Irritable bowel syndrome

It may seem odd to include irritable bowel syndrome (IBS) in a book dealing with stomach problems.

The three symptoms most commonly associated with IBS are colicky bowel pain, wind (usually causing bloating) and either diarrhoea or constipation or some combination of the two. At first glance it is difficult to see what IBS has got to do with stomach problems.

But in reality the two have a great deal in common. In addition to the typical large bowel symptoms which cause so much distress and discomfort, IBS sufferers often also complain of stomach problems such as indigestion, heartburn, flatulence and so on.

And these two groups of symptoms are closely linked.

When the bowel is full of wind (because of irritable bowel syndrome) there is, inevitably, a great deal of back pressure on the stomach. And that's what often causes indigestion, heartburn, flatulence and other stomach problems. I strongly suspect that IBS is now one of the commonest primary causes of these stomach disorders.

Although IBS has been around for a long time it hasn't always been known by the same name. Until relatively recently the symptoms which characterise this disorder were known as 'spastic colon'.

Irritable bowel syndrome is one of the commonest and most troublesome of all diseases. At one time or another as many as one in three people suffer from it. It affects men as much as women – although it is usually regarded as a disease which primarily affects young women in their twenties, thirties and forties – and it affects the young as much as the old. Children under ten can get it and there are many sufferers in their seventies and eighties.

I have no doubt that IBS is also one of the most commonly misdiagnosed of all diseases – and one of the most badly treated. Once it has developed it hardly ever disappears completely.

That's the bad news.

The good news is twofold.

First, irritable bowel syndrome is not, by itself, dangerous or life threatening; it doesn't turn into anything more serious, it won't turn into cancer and it won't kill you or even threaten your life.

And second, although it does tend to hang around – once you have got it you've probably got it for life – irritable bowel syndrome, or IBS, can be controlled. There is no quick, simple, reliable cure because there is no clearly defined cause. But although you may not be able to make the symptoms of irritable bowel syndrome disappear for ever – you can control it. Many readers have written to tell me that the advice I'm going to give you has worked.

Before I go any further I should deal with the symptoms of IBS.

First, there are the primary symptoms which involve the bowel itself and what goes on inside it. Pain is probably the most obvious of these symptoms – though it is also one of the most variable. It is often a colicky, spasmodic sort of pain which comes and goes in waves; it can affect just about any part of the abdomen and it frequently fades a little when the sufferer goes to the toilet.

Most sufferers complain of diarrhoea – which can sometimes be quite sudden and explosive – but, oddly enough, constipation is also a common symptom. Sometimes the two problems alternate.

The third very common bowel problem associated with this complaint is wind and this really is typical. Most sufferers complain that their tummies swell up so much that their clothes don't fit them properly. Many complain of embarrassing rumblings and gurglings and other noises and of the social problems associated with escaping wind.

Most IBS patients have these three problems.

Next, there are the secondary symptoms which affect a lot of sufferers but which don't affect all patients. If you have IBS you're almost certain to have the three primary symptoms but you are unlikely to have all of the secondary symptoms.

One or two of the secondary symptoms are caused by the wind that is so widely associated with irritable bowel syndrome and these will probably come and go as the wind comes and goes. Symptoms in this category include a feeling of being full all the time and of not being able to eat very much plus a constant feeling of nausea, heartburn and indigestion. Back pains of one sort or another are also fairly commonplace and these too are frequently a result of wind accumulating in the intestines. It's even quite common for irritable bowel syndrome sufferers to complain of urinary frequency and other bladder problems caused by pressure produced by wind in the intestines.

Last, but certainly not least, there are the mental symptoms which aren't in any direct way related to the intestines or what is going on inside them. Anxiety, depression and irritability are all common but the one mental symptom that really seems to affect irritable bowel syndrome patients more than any other is tiredness.

Even though you may be quite convinced that you are suffering from irritable bowel syndrome you shouldn't make the diagnosis by yourself without visiting your doctor. Although IBS is probably the commonest of all bowel problems today there are other problems which can cause bowel symptoms and only by visiting your doctor can you be absolutely sure that you have got the diagnosis right.

What causes IBS?

There are, as there are with stomach problems, two main causes.

The first is stress.

I know that the word 'stress' has been used a lot in the last few years. And you may feel that it has been overworked. But the plain fact is that all muscles can be tightened up when you are under too much stress. Tension headaches are a good example of what happens when the muscles around your head are tightened by worry and anxiety. The muscles in your bowel walls are no exception – they are as vulnerable and as susceptible to stress as any other muscles – and in some individuals it is these muscles which suffer first when stress starts to get out of control. Lots of people who don't suffer from irritable bowel syndrome do get diarrhoea or cramping pains in their tummies when they are under too much pressure or when they are anxious.

The second explanation for the current epidemic of irritable bowel syndrome lies in the type of food we tend to eat these days.

Most of us tend to eat a bland, over-refined diet that contains very little natural roughage. And our bowels can't cope very well with this. (There is more about IBS in my book *Relief from IBS*, published by the European Medical Journal.)

Peptic ulcer

The terms peptic ulcer, gastric ulcer and duodenal ulcer are often used as though they are completely interchangeable. In fact, however, there are differences. A peptic ulcer is simply any ulcer in the upper part of the intestinal tract. The word 'peptic' is used as a synonym for digestion. A gastric ulcer, however, is one that is found in the stomach, while a duodenal ulcer is one that is found in the duodenum. The phrase peptic ulceration can be used to describe both a stomach ulcer or a duodenal ulcer.

Ulcers of all kinds result from an imbalance between the power of the secretions produced by the stomach and the resistance of the lining of the part of the intestine concerned.

Wind (flatulence and burping)

This problem is one of the commonest of all health problems – affecting well over half of the population. Doctors really don't understand much about it. And can't do much to deal with it.

The normal gastro-intestinal tract is said to contain between 100 and 200 millilitres of gas under normal circumstances. During an ordinary sort of day a normal individual will often produce 1 to 2 litres of gas. It is, therefore, quite obvious that there must be a tendency for wind to pass out of the gastro-intestinal tract at one end or the other. (Wind consists of 250 different gases. The study of flatulence is called flatology. The most astonishing fact about wind is that it is normal to 'break wind' at around 100 mph.)

Wind is produced within the gastro-intestinal tract as food is digested, and some foods are more likely than others to result in the production of large quantities of wind. Brussels sprouts and cabbage are fairly widely recognised as offending vegetables and beans, of course, have a tremendous reputation in this respect.

It is, however, important to understand that not all of the wind in the gastro-intestinal tract is a result of the normal digestive process.

Some of the wind that causes such embarrassing noises gets into the intestinal tract in the same way that food gets in: it is swallowed. People who chew gum, smoke cigarettes or eat too quickly will often swallow air as will those individuals who gulp in air as a nervous habit. Indeed, two thirds of the gas in your body is probably swallowed air.

You're likely to swallow too much air if you gulp hot drinks or sip drinks through a straw. Habits like sucking mints can also cause wind to accumulate. Fizzy drinks are an obvious cause of wind. Chewing with an open mouth, or talking with your mouth full also increases the likelihood of wind. Foods that are likely to cause wind include: beans, broccoli, Brussels sprouts, cabbage, raisins, bananas, popcorn, peanuts, onions, chocolate, coffee and milk.

PART FOUR

LOOK AFTER YOUR STOMACH: GENERAL REMEDIES

'Indigestion is charged by God with enforcing morality on the stomach.'
Victor Hugo (1802-1855) in *Les Misérables*

See your doctor

If you have persistent or recurrent pains (or other symptoms) you must obviously see your doctor straight away. Similarly you should seek medical advice if you have any other symptoms which may signify a lesion affecting any part of your gastro-intestinal tract. Symptoms which merit urgent attention include (but are not limited to): difficulty in swallowing; feeling full after small meals; a lump (which you may be able to see or feel) in your abdomen; persistent indigestion; a poor appetite; weight loss; vomiting blood or a substance which looks like coffee grounds; and tarry, black stools (this suggests that the stools may contain blood). You should also see your doctor as a matter of some urgency if you develop digestive symptoms while taking a prescription drug. For example, it is well known that pain killers and anti-inflammatory drugs (such as those prescribed for arthritis) may cause stomach problems.

71

I believe that anyone who has persistent or recurrent stomach symptoms should seek medical advice before trying to solve their problems themselves. I say this not only because it is often extremely difficult to differentiate between various types of stomach disorder, but because it is also sometimes very difficult to differentiate between stomach problems and other diseases. It is, for example, often extremely tricky to differentiate between angina, which is an early warning sign of heart trouble, and indigestion, which is a warning sign of stomach trouble. And although stomach cancer is less common than it used to be it still occurs. Like all cancers it can be treated far more effectively if it is found early than if it is found late.

Your doctor may be able to make a firm diagnosis almost immediately, but if he is uncertain as to the precise nature of your illness he will be able to organise the necessary investigations. The great majority of stomach X-rays and endoscopy examinations show no signs of any active lesions, but they do at least provide some comfort by eliminating the possibility of there being any serious disorder.

Differentiating between angina and indigestion, between indigestion and peptic ulceration, between gastritis and gastric carcinoma and between simple heartburn and serious oesophageal disease requires professional assistance. I believe that anyone who has any of the stomach symptoms I've described for more than five days, or who suffers from recurrent attacks of any symptom, needs medical advice. Persistent symptoms or severe pain obviously merit an immediate medical consultation.

Once he has made a diagnosis your doctor will usually offer some form of therapy. Unfortunately the type of treatment that doctors offer is usually designed only to deal with the symptoms rather than to affect the cause of the problem. Your doctor may be able to help clear up your stomach trouble, but there is a good chance that exactly the same symptoms will recur unless you are able to do something to help yourself.

CASE HISTORY 1: MR KENNEDY

Mr Kennedy lived with his wife in a small terraced house where they had spent the whole of their married life together. It was rather an old-fashioned house and since Mrs Kennedy didn't like the idea of having workmen wandering through knocking out bricks and generally creating havoc they didn't have any electricity or an indoor lavatory. Everyone else in the terrace had both but the Kennedys remained resolutely opposed to any such technical advances.

They both managed quite well without these conveniences and although I was their family doctor I only saw them very occasionally. They were proud, independent and generally quite healthy.

It was Mr Kennedy who came to see me to ask for a bottle of indigestion medicine. He explained that every night when he went to the lavatory after his evening meal he had a pain in his chest. He was quite convinced that the pain was caused by indigestion, but although he'd tried adjusting his eating habits he hadn't managed to eliminate the discomfort.

When I talked to him I discovered that the pain had only begun to bother him during the winter months and that it had been worst during a particularly cold spell when snow had remained on the ground for ten days or so. More questioning told me that he had never had any indigestion at any other time of day, and that he never got the pain unless he went out of doors.

Mr Kennedy had made a dangerous and incorrect assumption in guessing that his pain was due to indigestion. In fact it was an angina pain produced by his habit of taking exercise during the colder evening hours. It is well known that heart pain is exacerbated by cold weather since the cold has a constrictive effect on the blood vessels.

Once the diagnosis had been made I was able to offer useful and constructive advice. In fact it was very constructive advice because, among other things, I suggested that they have an indoor lavatory built at long last. When they finally did so the chest pains stopped.

That story ended happily, but it could easily have ended quite differently. If Mr Kennedy had continued to regard his pain as nothing more than indigestion, and had done nothing about it, he could quite well have had a heart attack one evening on his way to the lavatory.

CASE HISTORY 2: MR BLUNDELL

The other patient I want to describe, Mr Blundell, worked in a car factory as a machine operator. He came to see me in quite a state because he was totally convinced that he was getting heart pains.

Every morning he drove his car part of the way to the factory where he worked but because of the congestion in the works car park he had recently got into the habit of leaving his car in the driveway of a friend's house. The driveway was about half a mile from the factory but Mr Blundell found it quicker to walk that last half a mile than to park his car and then make his way into the factory.

He was developing his pains every morning as he began his walk to the factory, and he explained to me that he had put the pains down to heart trouble for the simple reason that he could think of no other possible explanation. In fact when I examined him I could find absolutely nothing wrong. His heart was in perfect condition, his arteries seemed perfectly patent and his blood pressure was quite normal for a man of his age.

The real explanation for Mr Blundell's pain was quite simple. When he parked his car in the driveway at his friend's house each day Mr Blundell popped his head into the kitchen to say 'hello'. And every day when he did that he had a bacon sandwich popped into his mouth. He didn't like refusing and he didn't like walking along the road with a bacon sandwich in his hand so he scoffed the sandwich rather hurriedly. And that gave him indigestion.

TESTS YOUR DOCTOR MAY ARRANGE

Once your family doctor has listened to your story he will be able to make a decision about whether or not further investigations are necessary. He may, for example, decide that you need to have a barium meal examination. This commonly performed test relies on the fact that barium that has been swallowed can be seen quite clearly on an X-ray outlining the inner walls of the stomach and duodenum. If there are any abnormalities in the stomach or duodenum lining the radiologist who studies the X-ray film will be able to spot them straight away. Alternatively, your doctor may decide to refer you to a local specialist for an endoscopy. In this test a flexible tube is pushed down the oesophagus and into the stomach. Through the tube the viewer can see inside the stomach and duodenum and may even be able to take photographs.

If any of the tests that are done suggest that there is any need for additional specialist advice, or for surgical intervention, then your doctor will obviously make the necessary arrangements. In the majority of cases, however, whether the tests are positive or negative, your doctor will probably feel able to offer treatment without specialist help. Whatever treatment he recommends you should ask if he objects to you starting your own programme of stress control. My view is that whatever the nature of your stomach problem stress will make it worse and stress control will help to make it better.

THE LIMITATIONS OF MEDICAL TREATMENT

The majority of medical and surgical treatments offered by doctors and surgeons to people suffering from stomach problems are designed to relieve their symptoms and cure their existing stomach troubles.

There is after all a very strong tradition within the medical profession that it is a doctor's job to make a specific diagnosis and to then offer a specific, prescribable solution. This ancient philosophy means that there is a tendency for practitioners to treat patients with indigestion or peptic ulcers with specific remedies for indigestion or peptic ulcers. The symptom gets treated and the cause remains undiscovered. The disease gets treated and the cause of the disease remains free to do damage again.

This tradition is supported and strengthened by the widely held feeling that anything offered as a solution which cannot be sugar-coated, put into a bottle and prescribed is at best dubious and at the very worst highly unprofessional. Although the hazards associated with tranquillisers are now well recognised, and the advantages associated with relaxation therapy and stress control widely accepted, there are still more medical practitioners prescribing tranquillisers than there are recommending relaxation.

To all that we must also add the fact that for strong historical reasons the relationship between doctors and patients is based very much on single consultations. Patients usually go to see doctors when they are ill and doctors usually get paid for offering advice and treatments. Only in some parts of ancient China were doctors paid to keep their patients well. With the relationship so strongly based on the individual consultation it is perhaps hardly surprising that many modern doctors still regard their prime function as the treatment of existing disease rather than the prevention of potential disorders.

It would be nice to think that this archaic attitude might one day be discarded, that doctors might be convinced that a medical approach which contains stronger elements of prevention is acceptable, and that members of the medical profession might perhaps be encouraged to offer their patients advice on how best to deal with pressures and pains without developing ulcers, indigestion and other problems.

Meanwhile, until that time comes (if ever) I recommend that patients should themselves think in terms of prevention rather than treatment, of helping themselves rather than relying on medical aid, and should aim for a long-term cure rather than a short-term solution. The doctor is a technician. He or she is there to help you deal with your immediate problem. For long-term good health – and a permanent solution – you must take control yourself. And that is what this book is for.

Rules for better eating habits:

You can do much to minimise the damage that your eating habits do to your stomach by following these simple rules.

EAT SLOWLY

People often stuff food into their mouths at an unbelievable rate when they are under stress. A medical friend of mine, with whom I worked in a hospital, used to be spooning up the last smear of custard while the rest of us were still finishing our soup. He always had indigestion afterwards and had to sit for half an hour to allow the pain to disappear.

Try and put small forkfuls into your mouth. Stuff huge amounts of food onto your fork and you'll end up failing to chew your food properly. Chewing is an essential part of the digestive process and the saliva in your mouth contains enzymes which help prepare your food for the secretions produced by the stomach.

Try to taste each mouthful of food that you eat. That way you're far less likely to eat unnecessarily or too quickly.

If you are a fast eater put down your knife and fork between mouthfuls. That will slow you down effectively.

CONCENTRATE ON WHAT YOU ARE DOING

Don't try eating while you're reading or watching television. A little mild and gentle conversation probably won't do much harm but you should concentrate as much as you can when you're eating. Only by concentrating on what you are doing will you be able to tell when your stomach is talking to you. And if you listen it will talk to you, and tell you when you're eating something that is going to upset you, or eating too much.

BE IN CHARGE OF YOUR OWN STOMACH

Don't let other people push you into eating when you aren't hungry or when you don't want a second helping. And do be prepared to leave food on the side of your plate if you've had enough to eat.

REST AFTER EATING

When you've finished a meal have a short rest. Give your stomach time to do its job before you start chasing around again. But don't lie down. You should not eat a large meal before you go to bed. Give your stomach an hour or two to digest food before you lie down.

FIND OUT WHAT UPSETS YOU

It's a good idea to keep a notebook in which you jot down the details of any foods or drinks which upset you. Anything which appears in your notebook (i.e. upsets you) more than once should disappear from your regular diet.

Try to find out what sort of foods upset your stomach most – and avoid them. Different people are affected by different foods, so it is impossible to offer a comprehensive list of foods to avoid but if you do have a 'weak' stomach it is likely that any of the foods on the following list will exacerbate your symptoms:

❖   All fried foods
❖   Strong tea or coffee
❖   Fizzy drinks
❖   Alcohol
❖   Fatty foods
❖   Spicy foods
❖   Pickles, curry, peppers, mustard
❖   Broad beans, Brussels sprouts, radishes and cucumber
❖   Unripe fruit
❖   Very hot or very cold fruits
❖   Coarse bread, biscuits or cereals
❖   Nuts or dried fruit
❖   Any tough food that can't be chewed easily

You do not have to avoid all these foods if you have stomach symptoms. But do be aware that these foods can cause problems. The important thing is to find out which foods upset you and avoid them. Do remember that when and how you eat probably affects your stomach more than what you eat.

LISTEN TO YOUR APPETITE CONTROL CENTRE

You can do a lot to look after your stomach and keep it healthy.

To begin with it is a good idea to learn to listen to your stomach and to get into the habit of eating when you are hungry rather than just because the clock tells you that it is time to eat.

You may not know it but you have an appetite control centre which is designed to control your eating habits quite accurately and which can make sure that you never get overweight or underweight. Your appetite control centre can even make sure that you eat the right mix of foods – so that your body obtains all the protein it needs and the right mix of vitamins and minerals.

A study published in America some years ago showed that when small children were allowed to choose what they ate from a range of simple, natural foods they selected balanced diets which were just as good in nutritional value as the carefully balanced ideal diets worked out by nutritional experts.

Another study published in America showed that young children automatically choose foods that enable them to avoid digestive upsets and constipation.

A third study, done on soldiers during the Second World War, showed that when allowed access to unlimited supplies of food, troops ate what their bodies needed according to the outside temperature and automatically chose an ideal mixture of protein, fat and carbohydrate.

Unfortunately, most of us have lost the art of listening to our own bodies and we tend to eat three meals a day whether we are hungry or not, stuffing our bodies with food not because we need it but because the clock says it is time to eat. In practice the stomach does not adapt well to huge meals taken at lengthy intervals and it can cope far more effectively with smaller meals taken at shorter intervals.

The existence of the appetite control centre in the brain was first identified in research work done by Dr Clara M Davis of Chicago in the 1920s. Dr Davis's initial aim was to find out whether newly weaned children could choose their own food and eat enough to stay alive, select a good balance of different types of food without being told what to eat, and pick foods designed to keep them healthy.

The children in Dr Davis's experiment chose excellent and well varied diets. Their growth rates, development and appearance were just as good as those of children who had been given foods selected by nutritionists. The children chose the right food – and just as important – ate them in the right quantities. And they stayed healthy.

Later Dr Davis reported that in an additional research

project she had studied 15 children for between six months and four and a half years and had come to the conclusion that they all were able to select a good variety of satisfying foods, ensuring that they ate neither too much nor too little. Their eating habits were, of course, unplanned and may have looked rather chaotic to the trained eye but none of the infants ever developed stomach-ache or became constipated. None of the children who were allowed to choose their own diets became chubby or fat.

The conclusion has to be that the presence of the appetite control centre means that if you listen to your body when it tells you what – and how much – you need to eat you will stay slim and well fed for life.

Despite the existence of this astonishing appetite control centre most of us do get fat, of course. We eat the wrong types of food. And we eat the wrong quantities. There are several reasons for this.

Some people eat because they are depressed or anxious or miserable. They eat because they are bored. And they don't stop eating when they are no longer hungry. They become overweight – or ill – because they have overridden their appetite control centres.

There is evidence that babies who are bottle fed are more likely to put on excess weight than babies who are breast fed. And, of course, fat babies often grow into fat children who then grow into fat adults.

The appetite control centre is directly controlled by the amount of sugar circulating in your blood and is designed to ensure that you eat what your body needs, when your body needs it and in the quantities required. Things go wrong because you ignore your appetite control centre and instead of eating according to your needs you eat according to behavioural patterns imposed on you by the society in which you live.

Our eating habits are usually established when we are

very small. We are taught to eat at mealtimes (whether or not we are hungry). We are told off if we don't clear up all the food on our plates (whether or not we need it). We learn bad habits and we learn to ignore our appetite control centre.

If you were bottle fed when you were a baby then the chances are that you started picking up bad habits before you could sit down at the table. One reason why bottle fed babies tend to get fatter than breast fed babies is that while it is impossible to see how much milk has been taken out of the breast (and, therefore, how much is left) it is all too easy to see exactly how much is left in the bottle. Anxious mothers tend to encourage their babies to empty the bottle even when their babies are no longer hungry. (In fact there is another device in the female breast to make sure that breast fed babies do not get overweight before their appetite control centre starts to function properly. The contents of breast milk change slightly when the mother's body decides that her baby has had enough to drink. This change in the constituents triggers the end of the baby's feeding response. Breasts are far more sophisticated than most of us realise.)

These distorted behavioural patterns all help to ensure that your appetite control centre is ignored and overruled. Your eating habits are controlled not by your body's genuine need for food but by a totally artificial conception of its requirements. By the time we reach adulthood most of us have learned to eat for all sorts of bizarre reasons. We have learned to eat when we are sad or lonely. We have learned to eat when we are happy or want to celebrate. We have learned to eat simply because it is an official mealtime and everyone else around us is eating. We eat what the advertising copywriters want us to eat and we eat it when the boss says we should eat it.

However, you can break all these bad habits. By nibbling instead of gorging you can allow your appetite control centre to re-establish itself.

DON'T EAT TOO MUCH

People who are overweight are prone to a whole range of diseases – including many intestinal problems.

How To Find Out If You Are Overweight

Try The Pinch Test

When doctors want to find out how much fat there is in someone's body they sometimes use specially designed calipers to do the measuring.

You can use a simple version of this technique yourself. The big advantage of it is that it will enable you to find out which parts of your body contain the most fat.

Just pick up a lump of flesh between your thumb and forefinger and see how much space it takes up. If you try this test with the flesh on the back of your hand you will see that there isn't much fat stored there. But if you try the same test around your waist you will probably find that it is a very different story. Fat deposits vary from site to site around your body.

When you use your thumb and forefinger for this test you are, of course, picking up two layers of skin and two layers of fat. (Since human skin is fairly thin you are effectively holding two thicknesses of body fat). So, in order to get an idea of the thickness of your body fat at that particular point on your body you have only to halve the distance between your thumb and your forefinger.

You can probably do this measuring yourself. Don't squeeze until it hurts. Just make sure that you have a firm hold on the flesh you want to measure. Then, using a ruler, measure the distance between the skin of your thumb and the skin of your forefinger.

You can do this test all over your body.

If you want to do this test to get an idea of whether or not you are generally fat then the best place for the test is probably the triceps muscle at the back of your upper arm. You can also try measuring the amount of body fat at your waist, on the back of your legs, on your thighs, hips and buttocks.

If the thickness of your skin and under skin fat exceeds half an inch then there is probably too much fat there. Since the 'pinch test' measures a double thickness of skin and fat this means that anything more than one inch thick means that you have too much fat.

If you can pinch more than an inch then you need to diet!

Try The Mirror Test
Take off all your clothes and stand naked in front of a full length mirror. You should be able to tell whether or not you are over-weight – and where the excess weight is – simply by looking at your reflection and being honest with yourself!

Try The Tape Measure Test
1. Measure your chest with a tape measure.
2. Measure your waist with a tape measure.
3. If your waist measurement exceeds your chest measurement then you are almost certainly carrying far too much fat around your waist.

Try The Ruler Test
1. Take off all your clothes.
2. Lie flat on your back.
3. Rest one end of a twelve inch ruler on the bottom edge of your rib cage and the other end on the top end of your pelvis. If the ruler lies firmly on bone (with no flesh touching it in the middle) then you don't have a fat tummy. If, however, the ruler bobs about (particularly if you breathe or laugh) then you probably need to lose weight – and your waist is probably one of the places where you have got most fat stored.

Try The Waist And Hip Test

Divide your waist measurement by your hip measurement.

If you are a woman and the answer is 0.85 or more then you need to lose weight.

If you are a man and the answer is 1.00 or more then you need to lose weight.

GIVE UP MEALS COMPLETELY

Eating three square meals a day is old-fashioned and bad for you. Mealtimes are not natural. They were invented because they just happen to fit in with the way most of us work and live. If you get most of your calories three times a day at fixed mealtimes then you are almost certain to end up overweight. Calories that aren't burnt up straight away will end up stuck on your hips. In addition, there is also no doubt that you will make yourself more prone to stomach problems. Regular meals are better for you than irregular meals and regular small meals are better than regular big meals. By eating regularly you'll be helping to mop up some of the acid in your stomach. If you eat irregularly the acid in your stomach will have nothing to get its teeth into.

We've lost the art of knowing when we've had enough to eat. Most of us make the mistake of always finishing the food on our plates because we've been trained that wasting food is wrong.

Your stomach will be much healthier (and far less likely to succumb to stress) if you re-establish control of your appetite control centre by eating when you feel hungry, stopping when you feel full – and nibbling smaller meals more frequently rather than stuffing yourself with large meals occasionally.

The healthy way to eat is to eat mini-meals – and to eat little and often. You probably think of it as nibbling. Marketing experts call it 'grazing' because it is the way that wild animals eat. Whatever you call, it eating numerous small meals is much better for you – in a number of ways – than eating just three big meals. If you nibble – instead of gorging yourself on three big meals a day – you will have lower cholesterol levels and be less likely to suffer from heart disease. And I think your stomach and your intestinal tract will be especially grateful to you.

All the available evidence clearly shows that if you eat mini-meals whenever you are hungry your body will burn up the calories you consume. By spreading your energy intake throughout the day you won't ever feel hungry or faint. And you will be far less likely to put on weight than someone who eats three square meals a day.

Meals are bad for you.

Most of us eat at fixed mealtimes. We eat at breakfast time, in the middle of the day and again in the evening. But as far as your body is concerned this is a bizarre, unnatural and thoroughly irrational way to eat. Your body doesn't just need food three times a day. It needs energy supplies all day long. By choosing to eat fixed meals you create problems for yourself.

When you eat at fixed mealtimes you eat whether you are hungry or not. Instead of obeying your body's inbuilt appetite control centre you eat because the clock shows that it is time to eat. Your body's internal appetite control can make sure that you never get fat – if only you let it. But eating meals at fixed mealtimes means that your natural appetite control centre doesn't get a chance to work properly.

When you eat at fixed mealtimes you tend to eat what is available, what you have prepared or what you have been given – whether you need it or not. It is easy to eat the wrong foods – and to eat too much.

Because you and your body know that it will be some hours before you eat another big meal there is a tendency to overeat. Your body then stores the excess food as fat so that you can live off the fatty stores while you are not eating. But because you probably nibble a little between meals your body will never need to burn up that stored fat – besides, your next fixed mealtime probably comes just before your body starts burning up those stored fat deposits.

Try to get into the habit of eating only when you are hungry. And remember that the mini-meal diet will work best if you leave between 60 to 90 minute gaps between mini-meals. The mini-meal diet won't just help you get slim. Eating mini-meals will also help you to live longer.

When you start eating mini-meals you will soon find that you are fussier about what you eat – and you will eat only what your body needs. By eating just what your body needs you will look younger, feel more energetic, feel sexier, avoid infections and diseases and live longer.

In Okinawa in Japan people eat just 40% less than other Japanese people – they also have lower rates of cancer, heart disease, diabetes and mental illness. And more people from Okinawa live to be 100 years old than from anywhere else in Japan.

Reducing your food intake will probably increase your life expectancy and reduce your susceptibility to illness.

But do remember: if you are going to start the mini-meal diet then you must stop eating meals. You can't eat mini-meals and ordinary meals as well.

You don't have to be unsociable and leave your family and friends to eat alone. If they want a meal sit down with them but just eat a snack.

CUT YOUR FAT CONSUMPTION

Modern food often contains far too much fat. Farmers frequently deliberately fatten up their animals for the very simple reason that they get paid by weight. A large, fat animal will be worth more than a slim, more muscular animal.

A fat rich diet is bad for you in a number of ways.

If you eat too much cholesterol there is a risk that your body's white cells – crucial warriors in your body's immune system defences – may be damaged. And if you have lots of fat in your blood that will also affect your body's ability to deal with infections. In a normal, healthy body white cells constantly patrol your blood vessels hunting out bacteria (and stray cancer cells). If your blood vessels are clogged with fat your white cells simply cannot move around effectively.

And although some fat is necessary too much fat in your diet can make it difficult for your digestive system to operate smoothly, effectively and without discomfort.

To this you must add the fact that animal fat is often contaminated with chemical residues – toxic and possibly carcinogenic residues of drugs consumed (accidentally or deliberately) by feeding animals. Eat too much of this type of fat and there is a possibility that you will dramatically increase your chances of developing cancer.

It is often difficult to find out how much fat there is in particular foods. And it is often terribly easy to eat foods which contain a lot of fat without realising it. This specially produced list which follows is designed to help solve that problem. It may contain a few surprises!

Remember that the figures on this list are only approximate figures intended to be used as a general guide. And remember that if you cook in additional fat the effective fat content of the food you are cooking will rise – often dramatically!

Governments often recommend that a healthy diet should contain no more than 30% fat. I think that figure is far too high (probably because a relatively high fat diet helps keep the food industry rich and happy). I believe that you should aim to have no more than 15-20% fat in your diet. If for some reason you need to follow a low fat diet you may wish to cut your consumption of fat to 10-15%. (There is more about fat – and other

foodstuffs – in my book *Food for Thought*, published by the European Medical Journal.)

To calculate the percentage of fat in foods which are not
on this list look at the calorie list on the package label and divide the number of calories obtained from fat by the total
number of calories; then multiply that total by 100 to obtain
the percentage.

Almonds 56%

Anchovies 20%

Anchovy, canned, drained 20%

Apple 1%

Apple juice 0%

Apple, baked 0%

Apricot 0%

Artichoke 0%

Asparagus 0%

Aubergine 0%

Avocado pear 22%

Bacon, back fried 44%

Bacon, back grilled 35%

Bacon, streaky 38%

Baked beans 1%

Banana 0%

Beans, green 0%

Beans, kidney 1%

Beans, lentils 0%

Beans, lima 0%

Beans, pinto 0%

Beef, minced 26%

Beef, roast 34%

Beef suet 95%

Beefburger 27%

Beer 0%

Beetroot 0%

Biscuits, chocolate digestives 24%

Biscuits, chocolate chip 20%

Biscuits, cream sandwich 26%

Biscuits, digestive 20%

Biscuits, macaroon 23%

Biscuits, plain 17%

Black pudding 25%

Blackberries 0%

Blackcurrant drink 0%

Blackcurrants 0%

Bran 6%

Bran flakes 2%

Bran wheat 5%

Brazil nuts 61%

Bread, brown 2%

Bread, Currant 8%

Bread, English muffin 2%

Bread, French stick 3%

Bread, granary 3%

Bread roll (white) 7%

Bread, rye 2%

Bread, soda 3%

Bread, wheatgerm 2%

Bread, white 2%

Bread, white, fried 32%
Bread, white, toasted 1%
Bread, wholemeal 3%
Broad beans 1%
Broccoli 0%
Brown sauce 0%
Brussels sprouts 0%
Butter 82%

Cabbage 0%
Carrot 0%
Cashew nuts, unsalted 46%
Cauliflower 0%
Caviar, black 16%
Celery 0%
Chapatti 1%
Cheese, Austrian smoked 22%
Cheese, Blue Brie 38%
Cheese, Boursin 42%
Cheese, Brie 27%
Cheese, Caerphilly 31%
Cheese, Camembert 23%
Cheese, Cheddar 33%
Cheese, Cheshire 31%
Cheese, Cottage (low fat) 2%
Cheese, Cream 47%
Cheese, Danish Blue 30%
Cheese, Double Gloucester 34%
Cheese, Edam 28%
Cheese, Emmenthal 30%
Cheese, Feta 20%
Cheese, Fromage Frais 7%
Cheese, Gorgonzola 34%
Cheese, Gouda 31%

Cheese, Gruyere 32%
Cheese, Lancashire 31%
Cheese, Leicester 34%
Cheese, Marscarpone 46%
Cheese, Mozarella 21%
Cheese, Parmesan 33%
Cheese, Roquefort 31%
Cheese, Stilton, blue 35%
Cheese, Stilton, white 31%
Cheese, Wensleydale 31%
Cherries 0%
Chestnuts 3%
Chick-peas 2%
Chicken, dark meat, no skin 6%
Chicken, light meat, no skin 5%
Chicken, roast 14%
Chicory 0%
Chilies 1%
Chinese leaves 0%
Chocolate bar, milk 30%
Chocolate bar, plain 30%
Chocolate bar with nuts 26%
Chocolate drink 6%
Chutney 0%
Cider 0%
Cockles, shelled 1%
Cocoa 20%
Coconut, shredded 35%
Cod, steamed 1%
Cod, grilled 1%
Cod fillet in batter 10%
Cod's roe 4%
Coffee 0%
Cola drink 0%

Coleslaw 5%
Coley, raw 1%
Corn, canned, cream style 1%
Corn, canned 1%
Corn on the cob, fresh 0%
Cornflakes 1%
Corned beef 33%
Courgettes 0%
Crabmeat 5%
Cranberry sauce 0%
Cream, aerosol spray 32%
Cream, clotted 64%
Cream, double 48%
Cream, Fraiche, Half fat 10%
Cream, Fraiche 27%
Cream, half cream 14%
Cream, single 20%
Cream, sour 20%
Cream, whipping 39%
Cream crackers 16%
Crispbread 2%
Crumpet 1%
Cucumber 0%
Custard 4%

Danish pastry 26%
Dates, dried 1%
Duck, roasted without skin 10%
Duck's egg 14%

Egg, boiled 11%
Egg, fried 19%
Egg, omelette 16%
Figs, dried 0%

Figs, fresh 0%
Fish cakes (fried) 11%
Fish fingers (fried) 13%
Fish paste 10%
Flour, white 1%
Flour, wholemeal 2%

Gammon rasher 12%
Garlic 0%
Gin, whisky, vodka, brandy 0%
Ginger ale 0%
Goat's milk 5%
Golden syrup 0%
Goose 22%
Gooseberries 0%
Grapefruit 0%
Grapefruit juice, unsweetened 0%
Grapes, black 0%
Grapes, white 0%
Gravy (meat juices, fat, flour and stock) 9%

Haddock fillet, smoked 1%
Halibut, steamed 16%
Ham 26%
Hazel nuts 36%
Herring, grilled 13%
Herring, pickled 18%
Herring, raw 18%
Herring, rollmop 10%
Honey 0%
Horseradish sauce 8%
Hot dog sausages 25%

Ice cream 16%
Jam 0%
Jelly 0%

Kidney, fried 6%
Kipper, baked 45%
Kipper, grilled 11%
Kiwi fruit 1%

Lager 0%
Lamb chop, grilled 22%
Lamb leg, roasted 24%
Lamb shoulder, roasted 29%
Lard 99%
Leeks 0%
Lemon 0%
Lemon curd 5%
Lemonade 0%
Lentils 1%
Lettuce 1%
Liver, lamb's, fried 14%
Liver, pig's, braised 8%
Lobster 3%
Low fat spread 40%
Luncheon meat 27%
Lychees 0%

Macadamia nuts 73%
Mackerel 11%
Mackerel flesh, raw 16%
Mackerel, fillet, smoked 13%
Malt loaf 3%
Malted milk drink 7%
Mandarin oranges 0%

Mango 0%
Margarine, low fat 40%
Margarine, very low fat 25%
Margarine, full fat, 81%
Marmalade 0%
Marrow 0%
Marzipan 25%
Mayonnaise 79%
Meat pie 24%
Melon, cantaloupe 0%
Melon, honey dew 0%
Milk, condensed 9%
Milk, evaporated 9%
Milk, fresh semi-skimmed 2%
Milk, fresh skimmed 1%
Milk, fresh whole 4%
Milk, skimmed, powder 1%
Mince pie 21%
Mincemeat 4%
Mints 1%
Mixed vegetables (frozen) 0%
Molasses 0%
Mousse (fruit) 7%
Muesli 8%
Mushrooms, fried 22%
Mushrooms, raw 1%
Mussels 2%
Mustard and cress 0%
Mustard 8%

Nectarine 0%
Noodles, egg 2%

Oil, coconut 97%

Oil, corn 97%
Oil, olive 96%
Oil, peanut 96%
Oil, soybean 97%
Oil, sunflower 97%
Okra 0%
Olives (in brine) 11%
Onion, fried 33%
Onion, raw 0%
Orange 0%
Orange juice, unsweetened 0%
Orange squash 0%
Oysters 1%

Pancake 7%
Parsley 0%
Parsnips 0%
Passion fruit 0%
Pasta, boiled 1%
Peach, fresh 0%
Peaches, tinned 0%
Peanut butter 51%
Peanuts, salted 49%
Pear 0%
Peas, frozen 0%
Peas, tinned 0%
Pecans 74%
Pepper, green 0%
Pepper, red 0%
Pickle 0%
Pilchards 5%
Pineapple juice 0%
Pineapple, fresh 0%
Pineapple, tinned 0%

Pitta bread 1%
Plaice, steamed 2%
Plum 0%
Popcorn (no salt or fat) 5%
Pork chop 18%
Pork leg, roasted 32%
Pork pie 29%
Pork, spareribs 39%
Porridge with water 1%
Port 0%
Potatoes, boiled 0%
Potatoes, deep fried chips 40%
Potatoes, jacket 0%
Potatoes, oven chips 8%
Potatoes, roasted 5%
Potatoes, sweet, baked 0%
Prawns 2%
Prunes 1%

Quiche 28%

Rabbit 8%
Radishes 0%
Raisins 0%
Raspberries 0%
Ratatouille 6%
Red wine 0%
Rhubarb (stewed) 0%
Rice, brown, boiled 1%
Rice, white, boiled 0%
Runner beans 0%

Salad dressing: French 39%
Salad dressing: French low cal 4%

Salad dressing: Italian 60%
Salad dressing: Italian, low cal 5%
Salad dressing: mayonnaise, low calorie 12%
Salad dressing: mayonnaise: 75%
Salami 47%
Salmon, fresh 13%
Salmon, tinned 8%
Sardines 14%
Sausages, beef, grilled 21%
Sausages, pork, grilled 30%
Scampi 21%
Scotch egg 21%
Sesame seeds, dry, hulled 55%
Sherry 0%
Shortbread 26%
Smoked haddock 1%
Smoked salmon 4%
Soy sauce 1%
Soybean curd (tofu) 6%
Spinach 1%
Sponge pudding 16%
Spring greens 0%
Squid 1%
Steak, grilled 6%
Steak and kidney pie 21%
Steak pudding 12%
Stock cube 3%
Strawberries 0%
Stuffing, sage and onion 0%
Sugar, demerara 0%
Sugar, muscavado 0%
Sugar, white 0%
Sultanas 0%

Sunflower seeds 48%
Swede 0%
Sweet potato 1%
Sweetcorn 1%
Sweets, boiled 0%
Swiss roll 5%
Syrup, cane and maple 0%

Taco shell, fried tortilla 19%
Tangerine 0%
Taramasalata 46%
Tartar sauce 59%
Tea 0%
Tinned fruit salad 0%
Toffee apple 0%
Toffees 17%
Tomato, fried 6%
Tomato juice 0%
Tomato paste 0%
Tomato purée 0%
Tomato, raw 0%
Tomato soup 3%
Tomatoes, tinned 0%
Tonic water 0%
Treacle 0%
Tripe, stewed 4%
Trout 5%
Tuna fish tinned in oil 22%
Turkey, roast 10%
Turnip 0%

Veal 28%
Vegetable soup 1%
Venison 6%

Vinegar 0%
Walnuts 52%
Water biscuits 13%
Water chestnuts 1%
Watercress 0%
Watermelon 0%
White wine 0%
Whitebait 48%
Wine, dessert (port, madeira,

sweet sherry) 0%
Wine, table (burgundy, rose, white, dry sherry) 0%

Yam 0%
Yeast extract (Marmite) 0%
Yoghurt, fruit (low fat) 1%
Yoghurt, plain (low fat) 1%
Yoghurt, soya 2%

BUY ORGANIC FOOD WHENEVER POSSIBLE

In order to help keep your intestinal tract healthy I recommend that whenever possible you purchase organic produce which has been prepared without chemicals.

Nearly half of all the food sold in supermarkets and stores – including fruits, vegetables, bread and meat – contains potentially dangerous pesticide residues. Some chemicals are sprayed onto foods which have grown and which are being picked or shipped to the stores but many chemicals are absorbed when foods are growing and obviously cannot be removed by washing or scraping. Some of the chemicals used by modern farmers are known to cause cancer, asthma and a wide variety of other serious disorders.

Meat is contaminated partly because of the chemicals which are given to animals (to keep them 'healthy' and to make them grow more speedily) and partly because of the chemicals which are put into or onto the food they eat.

Organic food is grown without the use of artificial fertilizers and pesticides and the extra money you have to pay for such food is extremely well spent. Organic farmers use natural fertilisers (such as animal manure and seaweed) and rely on natural biological pest controllers, though some use natural plant-based pesticides.

Moreover organic farmers also grow crops in rotation so that their soil is kept in good condition. Growing the same crop year after year in the same massive field probably makes good commercial sense but it means that the food produced will probably be lower in nutritional value.

Organic food is more expensive than food grown with the aid of large quantities of chemicals simply because farmers who use artificial fertilisers and chemicals to kill bugs, insects and infections can produce bigger, more reliable, more uniform, more predictable and more attractive looking crops. Organic farmers, who have to rely on growing food the way nature intended, tend to have smaller crops and they are more likely to lose their crop through disease.

When buying food and looking for organic produce you should check labels carefully and make sure that you find good, reliable local suppliers. Many organic farmers sell their produce direct to the public and in cities there are now many shops (and even some supermarkets) selling organic produce, either as an alternative to food grown with the aid of chemicals or alongside such produce.

DRINK PLENTY OF FLUIDS

Most people drink far too little water. Try to cut down on alcohol, fizzy drinks and caffeinated teas and coffees – they can all make your intestinal problem worse. Instead you should drink six to eight decent sized glasses of water a day. If you can't bear the idea of drinking that much water look for drinks that contain no alcohol, no caffeine and no sugar or sodium. Herbal, fruit or mint teas are fine as are decaffeinated drinks. Alternatively you can try drinking pure fruit juice diluted with water.

I suggest you avoid tap water which may be polluted with chemicals and drug residues. Bottled drinking water isn't necessarily pure. Some 'spring water' has been purified or chemically treated while the stuff sold as 'table water' may be nothing more than filtered tap water. Try to buy 'natural mineral water' which comes from a protected, pure, unadulterated source and has not been tampered with. Natural mineral water may contain some bacteria (though not usually enough to do you any harm) and so you shouldn't keep bottled natural mineral water lying around once the bottle has been opened.

TRY TO LIMIT YOUR CONSUMPTION OF FOOD ADDITIVES

Food manufacturers use flavourings, preservatives and colourings to restore or improve the taste, texture or colour of the foods they sell.

Altogether they use several thousand different additives and in recent years there has been a considerable amount of discussion about the safety of these substances. Since the average consumer eats around 5.5lb (2.5kg) of additives every year the problem clearly could be a massive one. Additives enable manufacturers to debase foods in order to increase their own profits.

No one has the foggiest idea how safe food additives are but I honestly don't think anyone in power gives a stuff about this. I have in front of me a booklet which was published by a government agency. In this booklet the government sternly warns that 'ham and bacon couldn't be sold without the preservative that also gives them their pink colour' and claims that 'scientists and doctors who check safety evidence for the government are satisfied the use of these additives is safe'.

Feel better?

No, I thought not.

And you are right to be sceptical.

When bravely explaining the fact that flavourings are not controlled as tightly as other additives the same booklet boldly admits that this is because there are over 3,000 flavourings in use, in many different combinations.

So, there you have it.

One official reason for not controlling flavourings tightly is that there are too many of them to control properly.

My advice is to consume as few additives as you possibly can. Try to eat fresh food whenever possible and avoid buying pre-packed foods that are stuffed with chemicals.

The harm additives can do

Additives included in food can cause a massive variety of symptoms and diseases including stomach pains and intestinal disorders.

Many of the most commonly used additives have never been tested to see if they are safe for human consumption. Those working in the food industry excuse this bizarre fact by pointing out that there are several thousand additives in use and that testing procedures are lengthy, expensive and time consuming. I doubt if many consumers will take comfort from this.

I have heard some food company representatives defending the use of food additives by saying that only 1 in a 1000 people are likely to be adversely affected by a particular additive. I don't find that particularly comforting for 1 in 1000 is not good odds. If 1,000,000 eat a particular food then a 1 in 1,000 risk means that 1,000 people are going to be made ill by it.

I am also worried by the fact that many different additives are often used together. It is widely acknowledged that chemicals often interact. If you include two different chemical substances in one product then there is a real risk that the two will combine and produce something quite different. Modern foods contain so many different additives that it is quite easy to eat a meal which contains fifty different chemicals.

No one knows what all those additives are likely to do to your health. No one knows what long-term side effects may be building up. No one knows how those additives are likely to interact with one another.

Five tips to help you limit the number of additives you consume

1. In order to minimise your consumption of food additives I suggest that you try to buy as many fresh foods as you possibly can.

2. When you do buy processed or packaged foods try to buy products with a short list of additives. It is well worth remembering that the substance named first on the packet is usually the one that appears in the largest quantity inside the packet – other products should appear on the list in decreasing order of quantity.

3. Grow as much of your own food as you possibly can. Even if you only have a small garden you may be able to grow many of your own vegetables.

4. If you (or anyone in your family) develops new or unusual symptoms after eating a new product try to avoid that product in future.

5. Become a cynic when reading food advertisements and food labels. Over the last few years the food industry has managed to devalue the word 'natural' so that it has become virtually meaningless. For example, the phrase 'only natural ingredients' is sometimes used to describe foods which are stuffed with additives if those additives are chemicals that occur naturally, or synthetic versions of chemicals which occur naturally.

Don't drink too much alcohol

The liver isn't the only organ damaged by too much drinking. Stomach ulcers and indigestion are also common in alcoholics.

For men the weekly limit is 21 units spread throughout the week.

For women the weekly limit is 14 units spread throughout the week.

How much alcohol is there in your drink?

❖ 1 pint of ordinary strength beer or lager contains 2 units

❖ 1 pint of export beer or lager contains 2.5 units

❖ 1 pint of strong beer or lager contains 4 units

❖ 1 pint of extra strong beer or lager contains 5 units

❖ 1 pint of cider contains 3 units

❖ 1 pint of strong cider contains 4 units

❖ 1 average glass of wine contains 1 unit (pub measure)

❖ 1 average glass of sherry, port or vermouth contains 1 unit (pub measure)

❖ 1 average glass of liqueur contains 1 unit (pub measure)

❖ 1 single of spirits contains 1 unit (pub measure)

Give up smoking

Tobacco smoke irritates the lining of the stomach and makes it more vulnerable to attack by acid. All stomach sufferers will, therefore, suffer far less if they can give up smoking.

It can even help to keep away from air breathed out by other tobacco smokers. Breathing in second-hand tobacco smoke can be almost as bad for your health as smoking.

There are a great many different methods around which have been advocated as being suitable for helping smokers to kick the habit.

By and large any method that works is a good one. If, however, you've tried to give up smoking in the past and failed you might find it helpful to try one of the following techniques.

HERE ARE TEN PRACTICAL TIPS TO HELP YOU STOP SMOKING:

1. If you find the prospect of cutting out cigarettes in one brave move too much to contemplate then try preparing a plan whereby you have to cut out your smoking habit in easy stages. You might find that it helps if you begin by telling yourself that you won't smoke during mealtimes. Or that you won't smoke when you are working. Or that you won't smoke while watching television. This trick means that you don't have to produce such an enormous amount of will-power in order to reduce your smoking. Alternatively, make a list of all the places where you smoke (office, living room, bedroom, kitchen, car, train etc.). Put the list in order – with the place where you smoke most at the top. Now stop smoking at the place on the bottom of your list today. And each day work your way up your list – making a new place out of bounds. For example, start by cutting out smoking in the bedroom and the bathroom. Just tell yourself that you'll never smoke in those rooms again. And then add other rooms to your list as the days go by. Within a week you'll find yourself standing on the doorstep smoking furtive cigarettes. At that point most people find giving up cigarettes a positive relief.

2. Tell everyone you know that you are giving up smoking. Better still get them to sponsor you for your favourite charity. The longer you hold out the more money you collect – and the less likely you will be to start smoking again.

3. After getting your doctor's permission, take up very gentle exercise. When you realise how unfit smoking has made you then your incentive to give up will increase. But remember that before starting an exercise programme you must get your doctor's approval.

4. Keep a daily note of just how much money you spend on

cigarettes or tobacco. It is astonishing to see just how quickly the sums of money mount up. If you're cutting down on cigarettes keep another record of the amount of money that you've managed to save. You can reward yourself by planning to buy something you'd really like with the money that would otherwise have gone up in smoke. Put the money you save by not smoking into a jar and use it to buy yourself something special. If you're a regular smoker you'll be surprised at how much you save.

5. Imagine the sort of situation where you are most likely to light up a cigarette. Now imagine yourself coping without smoking. Build up your image of yourself as a non smoker and you won't need to smoke.

6. Buy a bead necklace or bracelet. When your fingers feel edgy without a cigarette between them keep them occupied playing with your beads.

7. Quit smoking with a friend. Ring one another up when you feel you are weakening.

8. Don't do anything else difficult while you are giving up. Don't diet, don't take on extra responsibilities at work and don't tackle other personal or professional problems. Make sure that you have all your mental strength available to help you to stop smoking.

9. Make yourself your favourite meals. Food will taste better when you stop smoking – take advantage of this.

10. Keep all your cigarette butts in a jar in front of you. The sight and smell will help reinforce your determination to stop. Alternatively try putting your nose an inch away from a full ashtray. Then take a deep breath. That is what you smell like to other people.

11. Here is a way to get your children to help you give up smoking: buy them (or, if you haven't got any of your own, the neighbour's children) water pistols. And tell them that they

can 'shoot' water at you every time they see you lighting up.

12. Try to make your cigarette buying as complicated as possible. Buy a different brand of cigarettes every day, for example, or buy cigarettes from a different shop. Never buy more than one packet at once. Buy in packets of ten.

Learn to deal with the stress in your life

It used to be said that individuals with stomach problems would get better quicker if they rested in bed for days at a time. I don't think that there was ever any real evidence that bed rest actually helped ease an ulcer or accelerated the natural healing process, and in fact I rather suspect that many individuals who were forced to rest in bed by dictatorial physicians may well have suffered more stress than if they had been allowed to remain mobile.

I remember that when I was working in a hospital one of the consultants used to insist that his patients with stomach disorders should remain in bed for at least seven days and preferably ten days. He also used to insist that no patients should be allowed access to the telephone on the grounds that any aggravation or outside pressure would simply make things worse.

I lost faith in this particular theory when we had a patient in the hospital who earned his living writing racing tips for one of the evening newspapers. He had acquired his peptic ulcer as a result of a lifetime of financial problems, and when he was told that he couldn't use the telephone to send his racing tips to his office, and that he had to stay in bed isolated from the television, the radio and the visitors who could bring him news of all the latest betting he got worse rather than better. Being stuck in bed and isolated from the outside world meant that he lost his job. The result of that was that his financial problems grew worse. And so did his peptic ulcer.

It isn't bed rest that helps – it's stress control.

GET TO KNOW YOURSELF!

In order to cope effectively with the stresses and strains which are today an integral part of life you must understand your own ambitions, fears and anxieties and you must learn a little about how you react to problems. Some self-awareness will make you far better equipped to cope with change and stress. Here are six ways in which you may be able to get to know yourself a little better!

First, what are your priorities?
Modern psychologists often use the word 'goals' to describe personal ambitions. It doesn't really matter what terminology you use, but it does matter that you understand your own priorities. What comes first in your life? Your job? Your home? Your family? Your hobby? Your friends? Is money more important than sex and is power more important than money to you?

Only by understanding your own priorities will you be able to make vital decisions quickly and wisely. If, for example, your boss tells you that you've got to attend a business meeting on the day that your daughter is in a school play for the very first time you'll have to make an important decision. You won't be able to make that decision unless you know precisely where your priorities lie. And you will find it far less stressful if you decide on your priorities in advance – instead of having to make vital decisions in a hurry.

Second, what are your faults?
The things we are most likely to complain about in other people are often the things we ourselves are guilty of. We unconsciously spot our own faults in other people; we hate in others that which we are ourselves most guilty of. So, for example, if you're always very upset by people who are inattentive when you're telling a story or anecdote then perhaps you ought to

consider whether you are always as attentive as you could be when others are telling you their favourite stories.

Third, are you more critical of yourself than you would be of others?

A patient of mine once worried herself into the operating theatre by imagining that her friends would all consider her heartless for having refused to have her elderly but vituperative mother-in-law to live with her.

After she'd had her operation I asked her whether she would have disapproved if any of her friends had refused to have *their* mothers-in-law to live with them. She admitted that she would have supported their decisions wholeheartedly. I pointed out that her friends almost certainly felt the same way towards her.

Fourth, what habits have you got?

Habits can be useful. For example, it's useful to get into the habit of cleaning your teeth regularly without having to remember to go and do it. But habits can also be annoying, harmful and a sign of excessive exposure to stress.

Habits can be annoying – because if you keep humming short snatches from the same tune you're likely to drive those around you quite insane.

And habits can be harmful – because if you stop at the pub every evening on the way home from work you're quite likely to develop a habit that you can't easily break.

Habits can be a sign of tension too. Floor-pacing, pencil-tapping, nail-chewing, ear-scratching, knuckle-cracking – all these are warning signs that there is a little bit too much stress around. If you can learn to be aware of these habits you can use them as a guide to the amount of stress you are under.

Fifth, do you blame others for your own shortcomings?

The workman who isn't very good will usually blame his tools. The housewife whose cooking skills are limited will often blame her oven. The golfer who spends most of his time looking for his balls will blame his clubs. The gardener whose seeds don't grow will blame the quality of his soil. We all do it; and when we're putting our blame onto some inanimate object it's probably a harmless enough way to get rid of our own feelings of inadequacy.

But when we put the blame for things we ourselves should or should not have done onto other people then things become rather more complicated. The shop manager who blames the counter-assistant for not telling him that he hadn't ordered any more supplies is probably being unfair. The man who blames his wife for not looking after the family finances more effectively may well feel inadequate for having failed to earn more money, or guilty for having spent so much on beer and cigarettes.

Blaming others unnecessarily can produce problems in a number of ways. The person who has been blamed may well feel resentful and that can contribute to a deterioration in your relationship with that individual. It won't matter too much if the individual concerned is one with whom you do not have a close relationship, but if he or she is someone close to you then this resentment can cause quite significant problems.

And even when the individual you've blamed isn't someone that you know well you may suffer from tremendous feelings of guilt afterwards.

Sixth, do you always yearn for yesterday?

Our society is an ever changing one and many people find it extremely difficult to accept that things will never be what they once were. But yearning for the good old days doesn't help anyone. If you spend your time wishing that life was as it used to be, then you're quite likely to become bitter and twisted and probably annoy those around you. Enjoy your memories but don't let them interfere with the present.

KNOW WHERE YOUR STRESS COMES FROM

In order to cope effectively with stress you must have some idea of what sort of things worry you the most.

Study the check list which follows and answer 'yes' or 'no' to each of the questions. Every question to which you have answered 'yes' indicates a possible source of stress.

Remember, however, that stress is by no means always bad for you and that life without stress is pretty tasteless and unappealing. You need some stress in your life, but it's all a question of balance.

❖ Do you wish you had more responsibility?

❖ Do you feel that you have too much responsibility?

❖ Do you hate your work?

❖ Do you feel that you are under too much pressure at work?

❖ Do you think that you are underpaid?

❖ Do you think that your workload is too great?

❖ Do you feel that you are unappreciated at work?

❖ Do you wish you obtained more satisfaction from your job?

❖ Do you feel that your prospects for promotion are poor?

❖ Do you worry about what will happen to you if you are promoted?

❖ Do you think that there are too many administrators where you work?

❖ Do you worry about the danger associated with the work you do?

- ❖ Do you dislike your working hours?
- ❖ Do you find your workplace unpleasant?
- ❖ Do you wish you had more pressure at work?
- ❖ Do you find it difficult to talk to anyone at work?
- ❖ Do you find the journey to work difficult or tiring?
- ❖ Do you think that your race or sex has affected your chances of success at work?
- ❖ Do you regularly skip lunch?
- ❖ Do you get home late from work regularly?
- ❖ Do you have to cancel holidays because of work?
- ❖ Do you take work home with you?
- ❖ Do you wish you had more friends?
- ❖ Do you ever feel lonely?
- ❖ Do you feel that getting married was a mistake?
- ❖ Do you buy things you don't really need just to impress the neighbours?
- ❖ Do you and your partner or parents have nightly arguments about which television channel to watch?
- ❖ Do you get annoyed by the noise your neighbours make?
- ❖ Do you wish you had a room of your own in which you could get a little peace and quiet occasionally?
- ❖ Do you find yourself always in a hurry?
- ❖ Do you sometimes feel that your children simply use you as a convenient servant?
- ❖ Do you find yourself having to be nice to people you dislike intensely?
- ❖ Do you sometimes wish you could get on a plane and get away from it all?
- ❖ Do you worry a lot about what other people think?
- ❖ Do you envy other people their material success?
- ❖ Do you always feel guilty if you do anything that you enjoy?
- ❖ Do you feel that you are a burden to those around you?

❖ Do you have to look after relatives who are a burden and a nuisance?

❖ Do you feel bitter about the way you are treated at home?

❖ Do you feel you have to change your car if a new model comes out?

❖ Do you have to telephone for a handyman if you buy a new appliance and it needs to have a plug fitted?

❖ Do you live in a house that you cannot really afford?

❖ Do you wish you had a hobby that you could really enjoy?

❖ Do you worry a lot about your health?

❖ Do you think you might have some serious disease?

❖ Do you regularly buy medicines for yourself?

This list is by no means comprehensive but it is designed to give you some idea of the sort of things that may be causing you stress.

There are, of course, no simple slick answers to many of the questions listed above. If you find your work dull and boring you may not be able to do anything to change that immediately.

But you may well be able to start some form of training programme that might enable you to get a better and more rewarding job in the future.

Or perhaps, if finding another job really is very unlikely, you could take up some hobby or leisure interest which would provide you with the sense of personal satisfaction that your job does not give.

One patient of mine who had a job he hated in a large factory grew prize-winning onions and had an national reputation for doing so. Another collected old maps, and although he found his job in the local planning department quite unsatisfying he gained a great deal of pleasure and pride from his hobby.

The important thing is that you should be aware of the

things in your life which cause the greatest amount of stress. Only when you have identified the particular problems which cause you most stress will you be able to deal effectively with those stresses and strains.

LEARN HOW TO DEAL WITH STRESS

One of the most effective ways to deal with stomach symptoms caused by stress is to learn how to relax your body and your mind. Minor stomach symptoms such as wind, indigestion, nausea and heartburn often get worse quite quickly and may continue for hours or even days if you make no attempt to protect yourself. Learn to relax at the first signs of any stomach trouble.

Many of the people I have met over the years have been slightly worried when I have suggested that they learn to relax. Some have immediately insisted that they could never do 'anything like that'. Others have looked at me with some concern, obviously suspecting that something must have got to me and turned me away from orthodox medicine and towards the 'fringe' world.

The great tragedy in all this is that a very effective form of therapy has been partly lost to many thousands of people because of this fear. The truth is that the various different forms of relaxation therapy which are available are known to work very well, and can often contribute a great deal to the health of those who are prepared to spend just a little time and effort learning how best to take advantage of these techniques. Research workers in institutions with solid scientific reputations have repeatedly shown the value of different forms of relaxation therapy, and their results have now been published in most of the world's leading medical and scientific journals.

For those who want to learn how to relax with the help of professional advisers there are many institutions and courses

available. Hypnosis, biofeedback, yoga and transcendental meditation are just four of the techniques which are used quite regularly by many professionals in order to help patients learn how
to relax.

However, I don't believe that it is necessary to join any
organisation, go anywhere or pay money in order to learn how
best to relax your body and your mind. I believe that you can
learn how to relax perfectly at home. And by relaxing you can
learn how to cope with stress more effectively and how to build
up your resistance to stress.

Before beginning to describe how best you can learn how
to relax I just want to point out that you must be prepared to
practise a little to start with. No one would expect to be able to
play a game of tennis or dance the tango without a little practice and exactly the same thing is true of relaxation. And just as
you will get better at golf or dancing the more you try it so will
you get better at relaxing if you continue to practise regularly.
Finally, the beauty of these techniques is that you cannot lose.
There are no side-effects – all you can do is benefit.

HOW TO RELAX YOUR BODY

When you are anxious, nervous or under stress in any way your
mind deliberately tenses up the muscles around your body. There
is a long established, sensible reason for this. By tensing up
muscles your mind is preparing your body for action; it assumes
that the best way to deal with the threat you are facing will be
physical action. Your mind is getting your body ready to fight
or to run away.

But most modern stresses cannot be dealt with by a physical response. You cannot fight a traffic jam and running away
from an electricity bill won't do you any good. Modern stresses
persist for long periods – and so muscles remain tense for long
periods too.

Learning how to avoid unnecessary stresses, how to build up your resistance to stress and how to improve your ability to cope with stress will all help you combat muscle tension.

But there is another, more direct way, to tackle muscle tension and the associated problems it produces: deliberately relaxing your tensed muscles.

Make sure that you will not be disturbed for at least twenty minutes then lie down somewhere quiet and comfortable and use this simple-to-learn technique to help relieve muscle tension. Don't do any of these exercises if you are in pain or discomfort. If any pain or discomfort develops while you are doing any of these exercises you should stop at once and consult your doctor immediately.

1. Take very deep, slow breaths. Stress will make you breathe more quickly than usual so soothe your mind – and your body – by deliberately taking slower, deeper breaths.
2. Clench your left hand as tightly as you can, making a fist with your fingers. Do it well and you will see the knuckles go white. If you now let your fist unfold you will feel the muscles relax. When your hand was clenched the muscles were tensed; unfolded the same muscles are relaxed. This is what you must do with the other muscle groups of your body.
3. Bend your left arm and try to make your left biceps muscle stand out as much as you can. Then relax it and let the muscles ease. When your arm is thoroughly relaxed let it lie loosely by your side.
4. Clench your right hand as tightly as you can, making a fist again with your fingers. When you let your fist unfold you will feel the muscles relax.
5. Now bend your right arm and make your right biceps muscle stand out as much as you can. Then relax it and let the muscles become relaxed. When your arm is thoroughly relaxed let it lie loosely by your side.

6. Tighten the muscles in your left foot. Curl your toes upwards. And then downwards. When your foot feels tense deliberately relax the muscles.

7. Tense the muscles of your left calf. You should be able to feel the muscles in the back of your left leg become firm and hard as you tense them. Bend your foot up towards you to help tighten the muscles. Then let the muscles relax.

8. Straighten your left leg and point your foot away from you. You will feel the muscles on the front of your left thigh tighten up – they should be firm right up to the top of your leg. Now relax those muscles and let your left leg lie loosely on the bed.

9. Tighten the muscles in your right foot. Curl your toes upwards. And then downwards. When your foot feels tense deliberately relax the muscles.

10. Tense the muscles of your right calf. You should be able to feel the muscles in the back of your right leg become firm and hard as you tense them. Bend your foot up towards you to help tighten the muscles. Then let the muscles relax.

11. Straighten your right leg and point your foot away from you. You will feel the muscles on the front of your right thigh tighten up – they should be firm right up to the top of your leg. Now relax those muscles and let your right leg lie loosely on the bed.

12. Lift yourself up by tightening your buttock muscles. You should be able to lift your body upwards by an inch or so. Then let your muscles fall loose again.

13. Tense and contract your abdominal muscles. Try to pull your abdominal wall as far in as possible. Then let go and allow your waist to reach its maximum circumference.

14. Tighten up the muscles of your chest. Take a big, deep breath in and hold it for as long as possible. Then, slowly, let it go.

15. Push your shoulders backwards as far as they will go, then

bring them forwards and inwards. Finally, shrug them high. Keep your head perfectly still and try to touch your ears with your shoulders. It will probably be impossible but try anyway. Then let your shoulders relax and ease.

16. Next tighten up the muscles of your back. Try to make yourself as tall as you can. Then let the muscles relax.

17. The muscles of your neck are next. Lift your head forwards. Turn your head first one way and then the other. Push your head backwards. Then let the muscles of your neck relax. Move your head around and make sure that your neck muscles are completely loose and easy.

18. Move your eyebrows upwards and then pull them down as far as they will go. Do this several times, making sure that you can feel the muscles tightening both when you move your eyebrows up and when you pull them down. Then let them relax.

19. Screw up your eyes as tightly as you can. Pretend that someone is trying to force your eyes open. Keep them shut tightly. Then, keeping your eyelids closed, let them relax.

20. Move your lower jaw around. Grit your teeth. Wrinkle your nose. Smile as wide as you can showing as many teeth as you can. Push your tongue out as far as it will go, push it firmly against the bottom of your mouth and then the top of your mouth before letting it lie easy and relaxed inside your mouth. Now let all your facial muscles becomes loose and relaxed.

How to relax your mind

Much of the damage caused by the stress in your life is produced not by reality – not by the real problems you have to face – but by your imagination.

You don't get indigestion because you are stuck in a traffic jam every morning. You get indigestion because your mind plays a fatal game of consequences and your body suffers. When you are stuck in the traffic jam your mind wanders about and plays with the possibilities: you're late for work, the boss is cross, you get sacked, you can't pay the bank what you owe on your house, you get thrown out into the street...and your life is in ruins. By the time you get to work your mind will have created a horrifying and destructive scenario. The traffic jam is merely the starting point: your mind does the damage.

Do not underestimate the power of your imagination. It is powerful enough to kill you.

But although your mind – and your imagination – can harm your health and turn simple stresses into major illnesses it is also possible to harness your imagination and to use the power of your mind to reduce your susceptibility to stress.

There are many ways in which you can learn to relax your mind and banish the problems and worries that cause you so much damage. But I believe that one of the very best ways to relax your mind is to learn how to daydream properly. Some of the purists who teach meditation professionally claim that to relax your mind properly you should aim at removing all thoughts from your conscious brain and attempt to replace those thoughts with a void. In other words, they believe that to relax your mind fully you shouldn't be thinking of anything at all.

Now although I recognise that this type of mental relaxation is extremely effective, I don't honestly believe that it is necessary to get rid of all mental processes in order to relax, and I rather suspect that most people will find it very difficult to get rid of all their thoughts. If you try it you'll see what I mean; you push out your worries about the holidays or about the car and they're just replaced by worries about the washing machine and the neighbours. Most of us find it extremely difficult not to think about anything.

It is, however, relatively easy to learn how to replace unpleasant, stressful thoughts with pleasant, relaxing thoughts and if you learn to do this then, in my view, you will be protecting yourself from the effects of those stressful thoughts just as effectively as if you'd emptied your mind completely.

Daydreaming is one of those valuable talents which most of us abandon when we grow up. As children we're pretty good at it but as we grow older it's a trick we lose. People complain when we daydream and eventually we begin to feel guilty if we sit or stand thinking about pleasant memories and not getting on with whatever it is we're supposed to be doing.

So it's something that most people have to re-learn. To begin with it is something that is probably easier to do in a calm quiet spot rather than somewhere busy where people are milling around and there are all sorts of distractions. I don't believe that there is anyone so busy that they can't grab a minute or two once or twice a day in order to practice a little daydreaming. The beauty of this simple technique is, of course, that you can practise it just about anywhere. A lot of people find the bathroom a perfect spot because they don't have to find an excuse for being alone for a few minutes.

It doesn't really matter what you think of when you are daydreaming as long as it's a pleasant memory and one that doesn't get you too excited. I must stress that there really is a difference between daydreaming and fantasising and that although a good strong sexual fantasy is very healthy it isn't necessarily the right sort of way to get rid of your tensions. If you spend your daydreaming time thinking about your favourite sex object you'll probably do your stomach more harm than good because powerful sex fantasies may be stressful rather than relaxing. For relaxation purposes you're much better off thinking about a peaceful day in the country, a gentle day on the beach or a good evening out at a quiet restaurant.

You can actually prove to yourself that your body is relaxing when you are daydreaming by measuring your pulse. Before you start relaxing feel and count your pulse for a full minute. Use the forefinger of your left hand and press it lightly against the radial artery which can be found in the area at the base of your right thumb. If you measure your pulse rate again when you've exchanged your worries about having just smashed the car for the third time in a week for a happy memory of a day spent soaking up the sun you should find that your pulse rate will have fallen.

With a little practice, of course, you should be able to daydream so effectively that you can hear the breeze rustling through the trees and feel the heat of the sun on your skin. With more practice you'll be able to daydream very success-fully in circumstances where there are all sorts of other distrac-tions. You should, for example, be able to daydream very com-fortably in a busy store, in a traffic queue or on a crowded train.

Learning to relax your mind – and harness your imagi-nation – isn't easy but it's no harder than learning to drive a car, learning to operate a video recorder, learning to dance or learn-ing to play golf. If you can manage to master one of those then you can learn how to relax your mind.

If you have ever watched a television film taken by a cam-era fitted inside a roller coaster car then you will know just how easily your mind can be misled and how your senses can fool your imagination.

As the roller coaster climbs and dives you can feel your stomach churning and your last meal struggling to escape even though you are still sitting comfortably in your living room chair. Your body responds not to reality but to what it thinks is hap-pening.

Doctors and psychologists have been aware of this phe-nomenon for some time. When the film *Lawrence of Arabia* was shown on cinema screens a few years ago the sales of ice cream and cold drinks rocketed; the people watching the hot desert scenes all felt hot and needed to cool off by eating or drinking something chilly.

This doesn't only happen when you have a television or cinema picture to stimulate your mind.

Most of us are constantly creating images and scenarios for ourselves simply by thinking about things. Invariably we then respond to our created images and scenarios.

If you are worried that you are going to be made redundant then your body will respond to your fears. Your heart will beat faster, your blood pressure will go up and your muscles will become tense. You will develop a headache, not because you have been made redundant but because you have been thinking about being made redundant.

If you think that your mild stomach pains could be caused by cancer then your pains will get much worse. If a young girl thinks that her periods are always going to be painful then she will tense her muscles as each period approaches and it will be painful.

Exactly how your imagination manages to exert this remarkable power over your body is still something of a mystery. But to a large extent the 'how' is academic. The indisputable fact is that although we may not know exactly how the human mind works we know that it will respond to scenes it has imagined just as positively and as dramatically as it will respond to reality. You can use your imagination to help your body – and your mind – relax by deliberately creating peaceful, relaxing images in your mind.

For example, try this:

Close your eyes.

Imagine that you are lying on a warm, sunny beach. It is a day in midsummer and yet the beach is quite deserted. In the distance to your right and to your left there are one or two families scattered around and you can hear the sound of children playing. But there isn't anyone close to you and the noises are very distant. In front of you the waves are breaking gently on the soft sand and behind you a slight breeze rustles through the long grasses growing in the sand dunes.

High, high above you can hear the seagulls calling to one another as they circle overhead. They and the distant children are the only sounds that disturb the peace and tranquillity of the afternoon.

The most insistent sensation is that of warmth. The sand underneath you is warm and the sun is warm on your skin. You have oiled yourself carefully with sun lotion and you can smell it still. If you opened your eyes you would be able to see your skin glistening in the sunshine. But the sun is bright on your eyelids and you don't want to open your eyes just yet.

You lie there, quite still and peaceful, soaking up the sun and enjoying the afternoon warmth.

If you allow yourself to drift wholeheartedly into this daydream then you should feel your muscles relaxing and your whole body becoming more comfortable. Your heart beat will slow down and you will feel drowsy and content.

This sort of simple relaxation technique isn't difficult to learn. But it is an excellent way to combat stress and to defeat anxiety.

I suggest that you use my simple 'daydreaming' technique to help you.

Try This Daydream
Imagine.

It is a warm, sunny day in early summer. There isn't a cloud in the sky and there is a soft, gentle, delicate breeze in the air which stops the heat from burning and the day from being oppressive.

It is a perfect day and for a few minutes you can forget all your fears, anxieties and worries. You are on a private island; alone, content and away from all everyday pressures and stresses; safe for now from the one thousand and one demands which normally make life difficult and which sometimes make it unbearable. You are alone but not lonely. Around you the world is quiet but the silence is soothing. Occasionally, the breeze rustles the leaves in the nearby trees and in the distance you can hear insects in the grass, birds in the trees and the sound of the sea splashing onto the shore.

You are walking, slowly and effortlessly along a narrow country track. There are no cars, no people, no noises, no fumes and no rubbish on your island. You can take your time. You have all the time in the world.

On your left there is a hedgerow. On your right a lush, green meadow. At the base of the hedge there are primroses. In the meadow early poppies are already unfolding their pink-red petals and dancing lightly in the whispering breeze. You are at peace with yourself and with the world in this private and lovely place.

You walk on knowing that no one will ever find you or disturb you here. This is your personal world. No one else can come onto your island without your permission. No one can interrupt you or threaten you or make you sad while you are here. You know that whatever happens elsewhere you are safe here.

Slowly, your track begins to curve around to the left.

There is a slight incline too and you realise that you are heading down towards the sea. Your island is a small one and you can see the sea all around you. It is a deep, beautiful blue and it stretches away, unspoilt and unmarked as far as you can see.

As you head down the track you gradually become aware of the fact that you can hear a stream nearby. You stop for a moment, move slightly to your left, and look through the hedge so that you can see the stream. It is quite shallow but the water runs fast and is sparkling and crystal clear. The bed of the stream is made of small, pretty looking stones though a few larger rocks poke up above the surface of the water.

Further down and closer to the seashore the stream spreads out and becomes even shallower. Standing on the far side of the stream there are a dozen sturdy but old and gnarled trees. Beneath them, in the shade, there is a soft, inviting looking, mossy bank. You stand for a few more moments and stare at what seems to you to be the most beautiful and peaceful spot in the world. If you turn to your left you can see the stream, meandering down the gently sloping hillside of your island. If you turn to your right you can see where the stream trickles down, between rocks and across a stretch of soft, golden sand, to the sea.

Using half a dozen large, stepping stones you cross the stream, sit down on the mossy bank and rest your back against a tree.

It is like sitting in the most comfortable armchair ever designed. There is nowhere in the world quite so beautiful as your island and there is nowhere quite so peaceful as this spot where your island stream runs down into the sea. You rest, alone, content and silent. You feel comfortable, rested and happy.

When you close your eyes you can hear the clear water of the stream gurgling and bubbling over its rocky bed. In the distance you can hear the sea crashing rhythmically and majestically onto the rocks. Above you the breeze is rustling the leaves of the tree you are leaning up against.

You can feel the warmth of the sun filtering down through the leaves and your whole body feels relaxed. You love this peaceful spot.

You can stay here as long as you like. It is your island, your hideaway, your private escape from the real world. Here you can rest, untroubled by anxieties, stresses, pressures and worries.

And what makes this private place so very special is the fact that you can take it with you wherever you go. Your personal island will always be ready for you; will always welcome you and will always offer you peace and tranquillity. It never goes dark here. The sun never sets. It never goes cold. It never rains. This is your Camelot. This is your passport to peace, contentment and happiness.

LEARN TO ESCAPE

A patient of mine who had persistent indigestion once came to see me to ask how best he could deal with his problem. I knew that the main cause of his distress was the fact that he and his wife ran a small corner newspaper shop. They worked every day from about five-thirty in the morning to about eight in the evening. They worked on Saturdays and Sundays and on bank holidays as well. They hadn't had a holiday for years.

Knowing that this hard-working schedule was contributing a great deal to the indigestion I suggested that it might be a good idea if he and his wife took a few days away. I pointed out to him that the money he was making wasn't going to be much good if he wasn't around to enjoy spending it. Rather to my surprise my patient agreed to the suggestion. He came into the surgery four days later to ask me to sign his passport application form.

I didn't see him again for a month and then he came into the surgery looking very glum. I asked him what was the matter.

'I thought you said I'd feel better after the break,' he complained.

'Don't you?'

'I feel worse,' he moaned. 'I was glad to get back to the shop.'

'Where on earth did you go?' I asked him. 'What sort of holiday did you take?'

To my utter amazement my patient told me that he and his wife had decided that since they hadn't had a holiday for such a long time they would try to cram as much as they could into the fortnight they'd finally managed to grab away from their store. So they'd booked the car onto a cross-channel ferry, filled it with provisions and set off to drive around as much of Europe as they could cover in fourteen days. They'd eventually managed to criss-cross through France, Germany, Luxembourg, Holland, Austria, Belgium, Switzerland and Italy. They'd slept occasionally in small hotels and once or twice in their car. They'd covered an average of just over 480 kilometres (300 miles) a day and they'd arrived home totally exhausted.

The shopkeeper honestly didn't seem to understand that what he and his wife really needed was a good old-fashioned holiday where they could wander around aimlessly for hours at a time, where they could lie in bed a little later than usual, where they could spoil themselves, enjoy themselves, get to know one another again and generally relax.

PLAN AHEAD!

Few things are more stressful than the things we don't expect. Sudden crises, disasters of any kind and unforeseen accidents can all cause a great deal of stress or illness. And yet many of the problems which do cause us great distress and which seem to be unforeseeable are in fact preventable. If only we could learn to plan ahead a little more then we would all be able to minimise our exposure to stress.

So, try to plan your life. Be aware that unexpected events and unforeseen pressures do the most amount of damage. If you can organise the way you live so that you are exposed to a limited number of sudden crises then you will be helping to protect yourself against stress.

Being organised minimises stress.

I remember, when I visited a casualty department at one busy general hospital, being amazed at just how rarely were there any real crises. There were many very ill patients being brought into the department and many potential crises. But things were organised so well and planned so carefully that in practice most of those potential crises could be treated as fairly routine problems.

I spent some time one day watching how the casualty sister in charge of the department made sure that everything was always well prepared for future crises. Whenever the department was quiet, for example, she would send two nurses around every cupboard and every cubicle to check that the supplies of syringes, needles and drugs were kept fully stocked. She regularly tested all the electrical equipment to make sure that everything was working. And pieces of equipment that were really vital were duplicated. There were, for example, two defibrillators in the resuscitation room.

At another hospital I visited things were very different. There the sister in charge was really quite disorganised, and whenever an emergency was brought into the department there was quite a panic as people rushed around looking for the bits and pieces of equipment that they needed.

Someone would discover that a stethoscope had been borrowed. And then it would turn out that the electrocardiograph machine wasn't working because the plug had been taken off and put onto the fridge. There wouldn't be a syringe of the right size available, and a nurse would have to be dispatched at top speed to another part of the hospital.

The result was that when there was an emergency everyone panicked. And, not only was the unfortunate patient not treated anywhere near as well as a patient in a well-organised department, but the staff found themselves suffering from a great deal of unnecessary stress as well.

We can all benefit from the example set by that well-organised casualty sister and we can all organise our lives much better than we do. Writing things down in a notebook is a good start since few of us have perfect memories. Most of us benefit if we have a written list to jog our memories from time to time.

It's also a good idea to keep letters, bills, receipts and so on properly filed. Struggling to find the right piece of paper may not sound too much of a problem but if you have to do it regularly it can add extra stress to your life. If you don't want to buy a filing cabinet then put your papers into large, old brown envelopes and simply write a description of the contents on the outside of each envelope.

When you're planning some special event keep a master plan and a special diary in which you mark off details of the dates by which time all the various problems need to have been solved. That way you won't suddenly find that you've organised a wonderful party but forgotten to send out the invitations.

It is also a good idea to learn to cope with minor problems in and around the home. It is becoming increasingly difficult to get hold of doctors, handymen and repairmen of all kinds.

And it is also worth preparing for the almost inevitable breakdown of the electricity or gas supply at some time in the next twelve months. Buy a spare lamp or some candles and try to obtain some form of alternative heating and cooking.

If you can avoid these possibly minor and probably temporary inconveniences by planning ahead then you will be helping to limit your own exposure to stress.

TRY TO LIMIT YOUR EXPOSURE TO STRESS

From what is known about the development of stomach ulcers, indigestion and other gastric problems it is reasonable to assert that the best way to protect yourself from future stomach disorders is to limit your exposure to stress or to improve your capacity to cope with stress. Stress is known to cause and exacerbate many stomach lesions. By limiting your exposure to stress or by 'stress-proofing' your body you will be able to provide yourself with some permanent protection against a stress-induced stomach problem.

In order to protect yourself against the ravages of stress you must first learn something about the pressures in your life. You must understand precisely what sort of problems are likely to give you the greatest amount of distress and you must try to understand the sort of circumstances in which you are most likely to find yourself exposed to damaging stress.

Once you have succeeded in identifying the most damaging stresses in your life then you must attempt to limit your involvement in outside affairs so that the damage done to your body is kept to a minimum. It is also important that you do not allow other people to put you under pressure by making excessive demands on you.

Finally, as I have already pointed out, you should also make sure that if you are planning any change in one of the four cornerstones of your life – family, work, friends and leisure – the other cornerstones are allowed to remain relatively undisturbed. If you make changes in all these areas at the same time then you will be putting yourself under an extraordinary amount of stress.

DON'T BOTTLE UP YOUR EMOTIONS

Improve your mental capacity to cope with stress by letting your emotions show. Don't try to bottle up everything, for if you do you will eventually find yourself unable to cope with even fairly minor problems.

However capable we may think ourselves to be each one of us has a trigger point, and the wisest way to avoid encountering any problems as a result of exposure to stress is to try and ensure that your daily level of exposure to stress is kept within your own personal limit. If you bottle up your emotions and refuse to let those around you see when you are sad or angry then you will be storing up your stresses and reducing your natural capacity to deal with the unexpected.

There are two important ways in which you can relieve yourself of your stored emotions without actually telling the people around you exactly what you think about them and without pouring a glass of water over the boss's head.

The first thing you should do is to learn to cry when you are sad. Tears are an important safety valve and an acknowledgement that you have reached crisis point. They provide instant relief from frustration and are a sign that you have accepted your own distress.

Boys are sometimes taught that it is unmanly to cry. This is nonsense. Tears can be a sign of strength not weakness. And after the tears there should come a time of calm and peaceful sleep. Tears can be an essential part of your stress control programme.

The second way in which you can get rid of those bottled up emotions is by learning to express your feelings of aggression in a relatively harmless way. And there are lots of ways in which you can do just that.

I once read with great joy of a fairly senior official attending an international meeting who was so exasperated by his colleagues that he walked out of the meeting, crossed the road, went into a funfair and proceeded to throw wooden balls at china plates until he'd got rid of all his tension. I thought that was a truly marvellous way to deal with an impending crisis, for smashing china is a really pleasing way of relieving tension and getting rid of aggressive feelings.

The Greeks do it particularly well – they love smashing plates during a good evening out in a restaurant. Just make sure that neither you nor anyone else can get hurt when you do it.

Showing aggression in this sort of way is sometimes said to be immature. I don't think it is. On the contrary, I think it is a sign of maturity and wisdom to be able to release your accumulated tensions in such a deliberate and sensible way.

BE PREPARED TO COMPLAIN

Don't be afraid to complain and do learn to regard bureaucratic institutions of all kinds with a healthy measure of disrespect.

There are few things more likely to produce stress than buying some much-wanted item, getting it home, taking it out of its box and finding out that it doesn't work. If that happens to you and the shop owner tells you that it isn't his problem now that you've bought it, let him know that you're not going to be fobbed off with any miserable excuse but that you're going to take your complaint right to the top.

That might make him change his mind but if it doesn't then do make sure that you complain. Write letters to the company which made the product and make sure that you get in touch with all the consumer protection agencies that could possibly be interested in your plight.

That way you may get a replacement, the company may try harder to ensure that the next customer is better satisfied and you'll probably be far less annoyed about the whole thing. If you're worried that you'll say something you might regret write a letter of complaint, keep it for 24 hours and see if you still feel the same about it then. Waiting 24 hours protects you against your own impetuosity, but at least you'll have been able to get some of your anger out of your system.

Take the same attitude towards officials of all kinds. They're employed to help make your life easier not harder. And if they don't seem to understand that, find a supervisor who does.

Start a regular exercise programme

The chances are pretty high that you aren't getting enough exercise.

You've probably meant to start exercising but have considered yourself too busy. Meanwhile, though you like to think you're fit you know you aren't. You may even worry that you're so unfit that taking up exercise could be dangerous. And there is some truth in that. If you suddenly throw yourself into a hectic exercise programme you could seriously injure yourself.

But not doing any exercise is even worse. Unless you exercise regularly your health will be at risk and you will be more prone to disorders as varied as arthritis, osteoporosis, heart disease and depression.

Most of us live fairly sedentary lives. We travel in motor cars, buses and trains and we use gadgets and machines to help us cut down the workload in the house and garden.

If you doubt me just count the number of hours you spend sitting down each day.

In a few thousand years' time we may well have adapted to our sedentary existence.

But at the moment our bodies are still designed for action.

Many of the diseases which are commonest today are partly caused by the fact that most of us do not exercise enough.

Digestive upsets of many kinds (including indigestion, irritable bowel syndrome and other digestive problems) can be caused by sitting around too much. These problems can often be made worse by not doing any exercise and made better by a well-thought-out exercise programme.

Regular exercise can help the human body stay young while growing old.

Exercise helps to keep the physical body in trim in many different ways. The heart and lungs and other organs work better when they are given an occasional work out.

Our bodies are built to be active and a sedentary existence will lead to premature decay. (I don't usually like analogies
which compare the human body to a machine. But if you leave
a motor car in the garage for several decades it will suffer. Any
structure which is designed and built to perform specific func-
tions will deteriorate if it is not allowed to perform those func-
tions from time to time.)

Stress, muscle tension and pain are interlinked, interde-
pendent and inextricable. If you are under stress your muscles
will be tense. If your muscles are tense they will feel painful.

The pain you get when you are under stress depends upon
which muscles are tensed. If the muscles around your head are
tensed then you may get a headache. If the muscles in your
back are tensed then you may get backache. If muscles inside
your body are tensed then you may develop intestinal problems.

Indeed, the relationship between pain, stress and muscle
tension works in other ways too. So, for example, if you are in
pain because of a physical injury you will tense your muscles.
As a result your susceptibility to stress will be increased.

Exercise helps to break up these vicious circles in several
ways.

First, when you commit yourself to exercise you deliberately put aside your daily worries and anxieties. By concentrating on what you are doing you force the stresses in your life into
the back of your mind – and both your mind and your body
benefit.

Second, by stretching your muscles exercise helps to remove accumulated tensions. As the tension goes so the pain
disappears too.

And third, many of the accumulated stresses in your body
are a result of frustrations and disappointments and uncom-
mitted anger. Modern life leads us into many situations where
we want to explode – but where we know that losing our tem-

per would be inappropriate or illegal. People who exercise regularly don't just get fitter, they also get rid of anger and aggression that might otherwise build up inside them. Accumulated anger is, of course, a major cause of stress related illnesses.

Our body's natural response to stress (which wants us to respond physically) leads to a build up of muscle tension. The change in your muscles is designed to enable you to fight or to run away. But usually you do neither. When you exercise your body you give yourself a chance to empty your muscles of those accumulated stresses and tensions.

Regular exercise encourages your body to produce soothing and healing hormones called endorphins – your body's own version of the opiates. These hormones will help heal your ills and make you feel better.

The result of all this is that a sensible, regular exercise programme which improves your general health and fitness will increase your resistance to stress and reduce your susceptibility to stress-related illnesses.

People who exercise regularly produce lower levels of adrenalin (a stress-related hormone) and experience less dramatic blood pressure and heart rate rises during ordinary types of everyday stress. As a result regular exercisers are far less likely to suffer from heart disease.

At the same time, argue some experts, the production of a chemical called norepinephrine (also known as noradrenaline) increases dramatically during and after exercise and helps combat depression, increase happiness levels and tackle stress.

The bottom line is that exercise is as important to mental health as it is to physical health. Walking and cycling can do your mind and spirit more good than lying flat on your back on a psychoanalyst's couch.

There are three main ways in which you can exercise your body and liberate your mind: aerobic exercise, stretching and weight-training. Because each discipline offers its own advantages I recommend that you use all three. I have prepared a stress-combating exercise schedule which I call Trirobics.

TRIROBICS DISCIPLINE 1: AEROBIC EXERCISE

Any human activity needs energy and your body gets its energy from food. But food by itself isn't enough – your body also needs oxygen to help burn up the food and to turn into energy.

Your body can store food but it can't store oxygen so when you are exercising, your fitness level – your ability to cope with enhanced demands or emergencies – depends upon your body's ability to draw in oxygen quickly enough to supply your muscles, organs and tissues when they are under pressure. Your lungs have to bring the oxygen in, your heart has to pump the blood containing the oxygen around your arteries, and your arterial and capillary system has to be well-developed so that the oxygen can get to the cells which need it as quickly as possible.

When you're resting your body won't have much difficulty in pulling enough oxygen. But if you are unfit then, as soon as you start to run or do anything physically demanding, you will get breathless, you will start noticing all sorts of uncomfortable aches and pains and you will become exhausted relatively quickly.

You may argue that you don't need to be fit because you spend most of your time sitting down at a desk, sitting in your car or slumped down in front of the TV set.

But you do need to be fit because your body was designed to be used and if it isn't used regularly then it will quickly start to deteriorate: your lungs won't work as efficiently, your heart will grow weak and flabby, your muscles will become weak and your circulatory system will stop working as well as it could. Your body's ability to deliver oxygen to the organs and muscles which need it will deteriorate and your body's capacity to cope with physical or mental emergencies will be dramatically reduced.

Remember, it isn't only physical dangers which put demands on your body. Mental problems – stresses and anxieties – also put demands on your body and if you are unfit then a little bit of stress will make you feel tired and ill and a lot of stress could seriously damage or even kill you.

The good news is that however unfit you have allowed yourself to become you can restore your body to physical fitness, and build up your endurance, by following the correct exercise programme (though, of course, you should see your doctor and get his permission before you start any exercise programme at all).

Jogging, running, cycling and dancing (and specifically designed 'aerobic' exercises) all exercise your heart and help remove tensions from your inner body – especially your cardiovascular system.

You should take part in aerobic exercise for a minimum of twenty minutes three times a week, but you should do so carefully. When aerobic exercise really became popular for the first time thousands of people injured themselves. Joint, bone and muscle injuries were commonplace. If you take care and follow my advice carefully the risk of injury will be minimised.

The right sort of exercises will help to improve the strength and efficiency of your heart, will increase the size and number of blood vessels capable of carrying oxygen around your body, will improve the tone of your muscles, will increase the efficiency of your lungs and will, in general, increase the efficiency of your body's oxygen supply system. In addition, as a bonus, you will find yourself better able to relax, better able to deal with stress, better able to sleep and better able to work hard without getting tired. You'll probably also feel more self confident and more self assured as you get fitter and stronger.

It is important to understand that short or undemanding exercises will not help build up your endurance.

If you get your exercise in short sprints you will get out of breath quickly – creating an oxygen need that your heart and lungs cannot possibly satisfy without forcing you to rest. If you get your exercise in gentle five minute walks you will never put your body under any pressure – and you will not improve your endurance fitness.

To build up your body's endurance capacity you must exercise regularly and consistently in such a way that your lungs and heart have to start working more efficiently and more effectively in order to get oxygen supplies to your tissues.

But you must not over do it. If you do too much endurance training there is a risk that you will put an excessive strain on your heart or that you will damage your joints.

When jogging first became popular a few years ago many enthusiasts spent hours pounding the streets and ended up in their local hospitals complaining of backache and hip, knee, ankle and foot problems.

The aim of any good endurance programme is to improve your general fitness levels – not to turn you into a physical wreck. The aim is to help you get fitter and stronger – so that you can cope more effectively with physical and mental stresses – not to turn you into a medal-winning athlete.

In order to build up your endurance levels the exercise you choose must demand oxygen and must result in an increase in your heart rate.

So much for theory.

Here are the practical guidelines which you must follow to build up your endurance levels:

1. You must undertake endurance exercise at least twice a week and no more than five times a week. Three times a week is ideal. It is best if you have a day's rest between exercise sessions.

2. Each endurance exercise segment should last for at least ten minutes. If your exercise segment is short then you should

be sweaty and slightly breathless by the time you have finished.

3. You can build up your own endurance exercise programme by studying the Endurance Choice Table which shows the value of different types of exercise. I suggest that you aim to score 100 points every week – accumulated in two or three separate sessions. To make things as simple as possible try to measure out (using a motor car or bicycle odometer) precise distances – e.g. 1, 2, or 3 miles.

4. Before starting an endurance exercise warm up your muscles and loosen your joints by exercising gently. And remember to cool down afterwards. You will benefit most if you perform warm up exercises that match the endurance exercise you are about to begin. For example, if you are about to start running then warm up by walking and then, when you have finished, cool down by walking.

Endurance Choice Table
1. Running
(out of doors on a flat course or on a running machine):

❖   1 mile in 20 minutes or less: 3 points
❖   1 mile in 15 minutes or less: 6 points
❖   1 mile in 12 minutes or less: 9 points
❖   1 mile in 10 minutes or less: 12 points
❖   1 mile in 8 minutes or less: 15 points

If you run for longer than 1 mile, work out your points from your time. So, if you cover 2 miles in 20 minutes you get 24 points (2 x 1 mile at 10 minutes per mile or 1 x 1 mile at 8 minutes per mile and 1 x 1 mile at 12 minutes per mile).

Note: If you are too tired to keep running don't be afraid to stop and walk. You can 'mix and match' walking and running and still collect points according to the schedule above.

2. Walking (on the flat):

❖ 1 mile in 20 minutes or less: 3 points (no points if walking slower than 3 m.p.h. unless you walk for more than an hour – e.g. playing golf – in which case you can score 5 points an hour)

You don't have to get hot and sweaty to improve your fitness or to get rid of stress. A gentle walk can provide you with enough beneficial exercise to reduce your chances of suffering from heart disease and to reduce your susceptibility to stress.

A study of golfers showed that just walking round a golf course three times a week is enough to reduce the amount of cholesterol in the blood stream and to help get rid of excess weight.

And the more you enjoy the exercise you choose to do – and the better you are able to forget your worries and anxieties – the more you will benefit from it.

To really benefit from your exercise walk as briskly as you can. Walking can protect your heart just as well as more energetic exercise such as jogging or playing tennis.

3. Swimming:

❖ 600 yards in 15 minutes or less: 15 points

4. Cycling (on the flat):

a) racing bike:
   ❖ 2 miles in 12 minutes or less: 3 points
   ❖ 2 miles in 8 minutes or less: 6 points
   ❖ 2 miles in 6 minutes or less: 9 points

b) mountain bike:
   ❖ 2 miles in 20 minutes or less: 3 points
   ❖ 2 miles in 14 minutes or less: 6 points
   ❖ 2 miles in 10 minutes or less: 9 points

5. Skipping:
❖   10 minutes skipping: 10 points

6. Aerobics class:
❖   Beginners' class: 60 minutes: 8 points
❖   Intermediate class: 60 minutes: 10 points
❖   Advanced class: 60 minutes: 15 points

If you attend an aerobics class make sure that it is 'low impact aerobics' rather than 'high impact aerobics'.

The difference is simple.

In 'low impact aerobics' you always keep one foot on the ground whereas in 'high impact aerobics' there is a lot of jumping and leaping about with both feet in the air – and an inevitable heavy impact when you land on the ground again.

The risk of developing a stress fracture or injuring yourself in some other way is much higher with high impact aerobics. One survey of 28 fitness centres showed that one in two people who attend high impact aerobics classes injure themselves.

You can build up your endurance levels just as well with low impact aerobics as with high impact aerobics.

7. Squash, tennis, football, rugby, basketball etc:
❖   60 minutes play : 15 points

TRIROBICS DISCIPLINE 2: STRETCHING

Flexibility is a major component of the trirobics programme. If you are too stiff you will not only find movement and exercise difficult or even painful but you will also dramatically increase your chances of suffering from injury, muscular pain and postural problems such as backache.

❖   If you spend all day at a desk your back muscles will stretch, your chest muscles will shorten and you will become permanently round shouldered.

❖ Women who wear high heeled shoes develop shortened Achilles' tendons at the back of the ankle. When walking or running in flat shoes they tend to suffer from strained tendons.

❖ Too much sitting results in shortening of the muscles on the back of the thighs – the hamstrings. Many cases of backache are caused by tight hamstrings.

Stretching helps get rid of specific muscle tension and also helps by extending your range of joint movement.

A few minutes a week spent stretching will improve your performance during the endurance exercise programme, improve your posture and general health and reduce your chances of suffering from a wide range of muscle and joint injuries.

Many people find that stretching exercises are mentally as well as physically soothing.

Simple flexibility enhancing exercises should be performed gently and carefully. Do not do anything that hurts you. And do not 'bounce' in an attempt to improve your reach or apparent flexibility. You will only benefit if you stretch slowly and gradually – and then hold the stretched position for a few moments.

Ask a qualified instructor at your local gym to show you some simple stretching exercises.

TRIROBICS DISCIPLINE 3: WEIGHT TRAINING

When you lift weights you won't just increase the strength and power of your muscles – you will also increase the strength of your bones.

Lifting weights will reduce your chances of developing stress related aches and strains. (As a by product it will also reduce your chances of suffering from weak bones or osteoporosis).

The aim is not to build up enormous amounts of muscle bulk but to build up muscle strength. You don't have to look like a weight lifter to benefit from weight lifting.

It used to be thought that weight training was of negligible health value – and of use only to individuals who wanted huge muscles. This isn't true. A study in Boston, US showed that after eight weeks of exercise ten frail ninety-year-olds almost doubled their muscle strength and substantially improved their mobility. Since muscle weakness is a contributory factor in many falls among the elderly, weight training could clearly prevent many potentially fatal accidents.

Most towns – even small ones – have well equipped gyms where you can (under supervision) learn how to use equipment designed to help you improve the strength of all your muscles.

My advice is that you should join a gym, or visit one regularly, and begin a varied but regular exercise programme. Ask a qualified instructor to show you exactly what to do. Exercises should be repeated. It is perfectly possible to get all the exercise you need in order to improve your physical fitness without ever going anywhere near a gym. But if there is a local gym I suggest that you join it. You'll benefit in several ways:

1. They are bound to have a wider range of equipment than you will want to buy for yourself.
2. Good gyms are staffed with well qualified instructors who can help you develop an exercise programme to suit your own personal needs.
3. You'll find that most gyms are friendly places. You will benefit enormously from the support and companionship of those around you. It is much more fun to exercise in a group than it is to exercise alone.

If you cannot join a gym the alternative is to buy a pair of dumb-bells. Seek advice from a skilled specialist on the best weight to use. You can use these to help you exercise and strengthen most of your muscles. When performing these exercises keep your head and body as still as you can. And, remember – do not do anything that hurts!

When you are holding the dumb-bells above your head or body make sure that you stop the exercise before you are too tired to lower the weights safely.

CHECK WITH YOUR DOCTOR

Before starting an exercise programme you must check with your doctor if you are in any doubt about your fitness to undertake an exercise programme.

Don't just rush down to your gym and start lifting the heaviest weights you can find or pedalling the exercise bicycle as fast as it will go – you'll almost certainly make yourself ill if you do. And you could kill yourself.

Try to find a gym with a good coach, a well run aerobics class or a sports club that you can join.

A good coach is vital: he or she will show you how to take your pulse before and after every exercise session. Within a few weeks you should notice that your pulse will go back to its normal rate quicker and quicker after exercising. You should also notice that your normal pulse rate gets lower as you get fitter.

Follow this advice:

1. Do check with your doctor before you start an exercise programme. Do not start an exercise programme until you have checked with your doctor that the programme is suitable for you. Make sure that you tell him/her about any treatment you are already receiving and about any symptoms from which you suffer.

2. You must stop exercising if you feel faint, dizzy, breathless or nauseated or if you notice any pain or if you feel unwell in any way. Get expert help immediately and do not start exercising again until you have been given the 'all clear' by

your doctor. It is a myth that you need to experience pain to benefit from exercise. Pain is your body's way of saying 'stop'. If you ignore a pain – or try to exercise through it – you will do yourself harm.

3. Do buy comfortable, well fitting shoes. It doesn't matter very much what else you wear when you exercise (though large breasted women will undoubtedly feel far more comfortable if they wear good sports bras, and joggers should choose clothing that prevents chafing and that enables them to be seen in traffic) but good shoes which absorb some of the damaging impact incurred on landing can dramatically reduce the risk of injury.

SET ASIDE TIME TO EXERCISE

Allocate time for exercise and stick to it. If you decide to exercise only when you've got a free moment you'll never do anything. You need to set aside time for a properly organised exercise programme. But it need not be much.

Three sessions a week will be plenty. You should allow a full hour for each session though to start with you probably won't be able to manage that much.

If you are really pushed for time you can squeeze a useful exercise programme into just three twenty minute sessions a week.

Try to make your exercise time inviolable and give it priority over other, less vital tasks.

THE MOST IMPORTANT RULE

Finally, remember the most important rule for exercise: it should never hurt. Pain is your body's way of saying STOP. If you ignore a pain – and attempt to blunder bravely through the pain barrier – you will almost certainly injure yourself. Exercise can be dangerous – particularly if you start a new exercise programme without planning your programme carefully and without thinking about the hazards. A badly organised exercise programme can do far more harm than good and can produce an enormous variety of physical problems – inevitably raising rather than reducing your stress levels.

PART FIVE

SPECIFIC, EFFECTIVE HOME REMEDIES AND TIPS TO HELP YOU CONQUER YOUR STOMACH PROBLEM

'About the middle of the night I was very ill – I think with eating and drinking too much – and I was forced to call the mayde, who pleased my wife and I in her running up and down so innocently in her smock.'

SAMUEL PEPYS (1633-1703) IN HIS DIARY

Coping with heartburn

Here are my top tips for dealing with heartburn. Do note that if your heartburn problem disappears then you can try going back to your old habits – but be careful.

1. Avoid coffee and tea.
2. Avoid fatty foods.
3. Avoid spicy foods.
4. Avoid chocolate.
5. Avoid peppermint.
6. Avoid drinks which are too hot or too cold.
7. Avoid alcohol.

8. Avoid fizzy drinks.

9. Don't lie down within three hours of eating a meal.

10. Try sleeping on an extra pillow.

11. Eat small meals.

12. Avoid unnecessary stress – and learn to deal with the unavoidable stresses in your life more effectively.

13. Anti-acid preparations will neutralise the acid in the stomach and provide a fairly instant relief. Liquid preparations coat the oesophagus effectively. The snag is that the stomach can react by producing more acid – meaning that the relief provided by the antacids can be short lived. The stomach is likely to respond to antacids in tablet form by producing a lower level of acidity – the result is that the desired effect may take more time but the effect should last longer.

14. Lose any excess weight.

15. Avoid tobacco smoke.

Coping with indigestion – 10 tips for sufferers

Most sufferers simply head straight for the bathroom cabinet or the local chemist's shop and take a few slugs from a bottle of white medicine. Traditional stomach remedies usually work well because they contain a substance which counteracts the powerful acid that is causing the pain. But swallowing a few gulps of antacid after your symptoms develop only provides an immediate and short term answer. There is a real risk that if you don't do something to stop your indigestion developing you will eventually end up with a stomach ulcer.

So, here are some tips on exactly how you can help deal with (or reduce your chances of developing) indigestion. Even if you're not already a sufferer you'll benefit by following this advice.

1. Remember that eating regular meals is better for you than going for long periods without food. If you eat regularly then the acid that accumulates in your stomach will have nothing to work on – except your stomach lining.

2. Eat slowly. Put down your knife and fork between mouthfuls – that should slow you down.

3. Put small amounts into your mouth. If you stuff huge amounts of food into your mouth then you'll swallow without chewing. Chewing is an essential part of the digestive process.

4. When you've finished a meal have a short rest. Give your stomach time to finish its job before you start chasing around again.

5. Don't read or watch TV while you're eating. If you concentrate on what you're doing when you have a meal then you'll be much more likely to know when you've had enough to eat. Overeating is a common cause of stomach problems.

6. Don't let other people push you into eating more than you want. Be prepared to leave food on the side of your plate if you've had enough.

7. Avoid any foods which upset your stomach. The sort of foods that can cause upsets are: all fried foods, fizzy drinks, alcohol, strong tea or coffee, fatty foods, spicy foods, unripe fruit, very hot or very cold foods, tough food that can't be chewed easily, pickles, sprouts, radishes, cucumber, coarse bread, biscuits or cereals, nuts and dried fruit.

8. Some people believe that drinking water with a meal dilutes the digestive juices and adversely affects digestion. This isn't true. Water (or wine) taken with a meal stimulates stomach acidity and triggers the digestive process in the small intestine. Sipping water with a meal should actually help the digestive process. (And if you really, really feel that drinking interferes with your digestion you should drink a glass

or two of water at room temperature half an hour before, not after, a meal.) Other drinks worth trying include fennel tea and peppermint tea.

9. Try charcoal tablets.

10. Eat honey. A spoonful of honey or a honey sandwich may help. I have no idea why. But it often does.

Finally, remember that tobacco smoke will irritate your stomach too.

If you suffer from recurrent or persistent indigestion (lasting more than five days) then you must see your doctor.

Coping with irritable bowel syndrome

Although I know of no single wonder cure for irritable bowel syndrome there are a good many ways in which you can help yourself. You will, of course, have visited your doctor and he may well be treating you. You should tell him if you decide to follow any of the advice which follows.

First, you should take a good, hard look at the amount of stress in your life.

Try, for example, to make a list of all the things which worry you, which make you feel uptight, which keep you awake at night, which give you butterflies in your stomach or which you know upset you.

Try to decide what things are really important to you. Decide how you are going to allocate your time. And make sure that every week you take some time off.

If you want to relax properly you're going to have to work at it – and that will take a little effort and a little time.

Next, you probably need to take a long, cool, careful and critical look at your diet.

You will almost certainly benefit if you gradually increase the amount of fibre that you eat. To do this start eating wholemeal bread or high bran cereals. Eat wholewheat pasta, brown rice, oats – in porridge for example – and more fresh vegetables and fruit. If you suffer a lot from wind you will probably be wise to avoid any vegetables – such as sprouts – which seem to cause you a lot of wind. Nibble fruit and nuts instead of chocolate and sweets and eat pulses – such as baked beans. (But be careful if they cause wind – which they may well do.)

Try to cut down your fat intake too.

If you eat meat then cut off the visible fat. Avoid red meats as often as you can. Drink skimmed or semi-skimmed milk rather than the full fat variety – though many IBS sufferers find that they benefit by cutting out dairy produce completely. Make low fat pastry, don't add fat when cooking and grill, bake, steam, poach, casserole and boil rather than roasting or frying.

You may find that it helps if you drink more fluids. Good, clean, pure water is the best drink.

Next, try to do more exercise – but do get your doctor's approval first. Don't make the mistake of adding stress to your life by trying to run faster than anyone else. But if your doctor approves try to take more exercise of they type that you enjoy. Walk, swim, dance, cycle or work out in the gym – all those things will help you because gentle, regular exercise seems to have a soothing effect on the bowel.

HERE ARE TWELVE THINGS EVERY IBS SUFFERER SHOULD KNOW

1. IBS affects three times as many women as men (though I have suspicion that this may be because men are reluctant to own up to these symptoms – or are more likely to gloss over them and blame them on drinking too much or eating unwisely).

2. IBS sufferers have an especially sensitive gastro-intestinal tract – sensitive to stress, food, drugs, hormones or any other irritations. These stimulants cause the gastro-intestinal tract

to contract abnormally and they also seem to increase the sensitivity of the pain receptors in the large intestine.

3. Contractions within the gastro-intestinal tract become stronger and more frequent during an attack of IBS – resulting in cramp like pains and diarrhoea.

4. The pains and discomfort of IBS only rarely wake a sufferer. They nearly always occur when an individual is awake.

5. A high fat diet may cause symptoms. Other causes (or aggravations) include dairy produce, coffee, tea, citrus fruits and wheat.

6. When IBS patients eat they sometimes develop periodic constipation or diarrhoea with pain. There may be mucus in the faeces. The 'spastic colon' pain often comes either as cramps or as continuous dull aching in the area of the lower abdomen. Bloating, anxiety, difficulty in concentrating, nausea, headaches and tiredness are other common symptoms. Opening the bowels often relieves the pain. Sometimes there is relatively little pain with IBS – just diarrhoea (sometimes sudden and urgent) or constipation.

7. There is often some tenderness over the lower part of the abdomen.

8. Avoid particular types of food or stress which trigger the problem.

9. Regular physical activity (gentle exercise) often helps.

10. Avoid foods such as cabbage which are difficult to digest.

11. Artificial sweeteners and fructose may cause problems. Some IBS sufferers benefit if they eat more fibre. Others (particularly those who suffer from flatulence or bloating) find that this makes things worse. Numerous drugs are prescribed for IBS. Their value seems to vary.

12. Three types of bacteria which may prove helpful are bifidobacteria, lactobacillus acidophilus and lactobacillus bulgaricus. These three may be helpful in creating a healthy bowel and can probably be best obtained by eating yoghurt.

(If you don't want to eat dairy produce you can eat soya yoghurt.) The three bacteria help digest proteins, help digest lactose, help keep the bowels mildly acidic (which keeps the bowel healthier), manufacture some useful vitamins (notably B and K vitamins), stimulate the contraction of the bowel walls and kill harmful organisms (thereby helping to prevent food poisoning and diarrhoea).

Coping with wind: tips for wind sufferers

1. Swallowing air is a common (and unconscious) cause of bloating.

2. Bacterial metabolism of food in the intestine may cause gas. Some foods – e.g. beans and cabbage – are worse than others.

3. Eating simple sugars may make wind worse. Foods to avoid in particular include table sugar, sweets, biscuits, cakes, crisps, white bread and processed breakfast cereals. Remember that around 80% of the sugar we eat annually comes from packaged foods.

4. Tolerance to the amount of gas in the intestine varies enormously. Some people are particularly sensitive to it.

5. Eating too quickly can result in air being swallowed. Chewing gum and smoking cigarettes can both result in more air being swallowed.

6. Drinking water can help reduce bloating. You need two to three litres a day. Coffee, tea and cola drinks don't count because they tend to make things worse. Try drinking fennel tea – it can be very effective. Peppermint tea may also help.

7. Wind sufferers should avoid the following foods: milk and dairy produce, fresh fruits, some vegetables. Carbonated beverages may make things worse – as may antacids such as baking soda.

8. Some people benefit by eating more fibre. Others benefit by eating less.

9. If the gas coming out smells unpleasant then you are probably eating too much animal protein (or failing to digest it properly). Animal proteins contain large amounts of sulphur – which smells a lot.

10. Too much fat encourages inflammation in the intestinal tract. And this can cause bloating.

11. The foods we are most likely to be sensitive to (and which are most likely to cause problems) are the foods to which we are addicted. So, if you can't stop eating chocolate you are probably sensitive to it. If cheese is your favourite food then you may well be sensitive to dairy produce.

***

AND FINALLY...

'Look to your health: and if you have it, praise God, and value it next to a good conscience; for health is the second blessing that we mortals are capable of; a blessing that money cannot buy.'
    IZAAK WALTON (1593-1683)

'Doctors are always working to preserve our health and cooks to destroy it, but the latter are the more often successful.'
    DENIS DIDEROT (1713-1784)

'Strive to preserve your health; and in this you will the better succeed in proportion as you keep clear of the physicians, for their drugs are a kind of alchemy concerning which there are no fewer books than there are medicines.'
    LEONARDO DA VINCI (1452-1519)

'...no road that would lead us to health is either arduous or expensive.'
    MICHEL DE MONTAIGNE (1533-1592)

'To preserve one's health by too strict a regime is in itself a tedious malady.'
    DUC FRANCOIS DE LA ROCHEFOUCAULD (1613-1680)

Vernon Coleman 2000

For a catalogue of Vernon Coleman's books
please write to:

Publishing House
Trinity Place
Barnstaple
Devon EX32 9HJ
England

Telephone	01271 328892
Fax	01271 328768

Outside the UK:

Telephone	+44 1271 328892
Fax	+44 1271 328768

Or visit our websites:

www.vernoncoleman.com
www.lookingforapresent.com
www.makeyourselfbetter.net

Relief from IBS

If you suffer from irritable bowel syndrome (IBS) you will know only too well just how much IBS can affect your life. Thousands of readers have already benefited from Vernon Coleman's advice in his book **Relief from IBS**.

The advice he gives is easy to follow and includes a series of simple, practical tips designed to help you deal with IBS effectively and permanently.

As with all Dr Coleman's books many readers have written to say how valuable they have found this book.

'I wish to thank you for your quite wonderful book which I fervently wish I had read years ago,' wrote J.C. of Port Erin.

'I've just finished your book on IBS and found it helpful and instructive,' wrote Mrs W of Devon

paperback £9.95

Published by European Medical Journal
Order from Publishing House • Trinity Place • Barnstaple •
Devon EX32 9HJ • England
Telephone 01271 328892 • Fax 01271 328768

How To Overcome Toxic Stress and the Twenty-First Century Blues

If you are frustrated, bored, lonely, angry, sad, tired, listless, frightened, unhappy or tearful then it is possible that you are suffering from Toxic Stress.

After three decades of research Dr Coleman has come up with his own antidote to Toxic Stress which he shares with you in this inspirational book. In order to feel well and happy again you need to take a close look at your life and put things back in the right order. Dr Coleman shows you how to value the worthwhile things in life and give less time to things which matter very little at all.

The book contains hundreds of practical tips on how to cope with the stresses and strains of daily life.

'*Never have I read a book that is so startlingly true. I was dumbfounded by your wisdom. You will go down in history as one of the truly great health reformers of our time*' (Extracted from a letter to the author)

'*This book is absolutely outstanding ... it addresses a serious problem which up until now has not been identified or discussed in any meaningful way. If you feel you have a lot of stress being generated from outside your life, this book is an absolute must. Personally, I am going to get five copies so that I can put them in my lending library and lend them to as many people as I can.*' (Health Consciousness, USA)

paperback £9.95

Published by European Medical Journal
Order from Publishing House • Trinity Place • Barnstaple •
Devon EX32 9HJ • England
Telephone 01271 328892 • Fax 01271 328768

Bodypower
The secret of self-healing

A new edition of the sensational book which hit the Sunday Times bestseller list and the Bookseller Top Ten Chart.
This international bestseller shows you how you can harness your body's amazing powers to help you cure 9 out of 10 illnesses without seeing a doctor!
The book also covers:

- How your personality affects your health
- How to stay slim for life
- How to break bad habits
- How to relax your body and mind
- How to improve your figure
- And much much more!

'*Don't miss it. Dr Coleman's theories could change your life*'
(Sunday Mirror)

'*A marvellously succinct and simple account of how the body can heal itself without resorting to drugs*'
(The Spectator)

'*Could make stress a thing of the past*'
(Woman's World)

paperback £9.95

Published by European Medical Journal
Order from Publishing House • Trinity Place • Barnstaple •
Devon EX32 9HJ • England
Telephone 01271 328892 • Fax 01271 328768

Mindpower

How to use your mind to heal your body

A new edition of this bestselling manual

- A new approach to health care
- How your mind influences your body
- How to control destructive emotions
- How to deal with guilt
- How to harness positive emotions
- How daydreaming can relax your mind
- How to use your personal strengths
- How to conquer your weaknesses
- How to teach yourself mental self defence
- Specific advice to help you enjoy good health
- and much, much more!

What they said about the first edition:

'*Dr Coleman explains the importance of mental attitude in controlling and treating illness, and suggests some easy-to-learn techniques.*'
(Woman's World)
'*An insight into the most powerful healing agent in the world – the power of the mind.*'
(Birmingham Post)
'*Based on an inspiring message of hope.*
(Western Morning News)
It will be another bestseller.'
(Nursing Times)

paperback £9.95

Published by European Medical Journal
Order from Publishing House • Trinity Place • Barnstaple •
Devon EX32 9HJ • England
Telephone 01271 328892 • Fax 01271 328768

Spiritpower

Discover your spiritual strength

- Find out who you are (and what you want)
- Three words that can change your life
- How to get what you want out of life
- Use your imagination and your subconscious mind
- Why you have more power than you think you have
- How you can control your own health
- Why you shouldn't be afraid to be a rebel
- How to stand up for yourself
- Know your fears and learn how to conquer them

What the papers say about Spiritpower:

'The final tome in his trilogy which has produced the bestsellers Bodypower and Mindpower, this is Dr Coleman's assessment of our current spiritual environment, and his prescriptions for change. He advises both awareness and rebellion, recommending ways to regain personal autonomy and fulfilment.' (The Good Book Guide)

'Spiritpower will show you how to find freedom and give meaning to your life.' (Scunthorpe Evening Telegraph)

'This is a handbook for tomorrow's revolutionaries. Dr Coleman offers an understanding of the society we live in, in order to show where our freedom was lost.' (Greenock Telegraph)

paperback £9.95

Published by European Medical Journal
Order from Publishing House • Trinity Place • Barnstaple •
Devon EX32 9HJ • England
Telephone 01271 328892 • Fax 01271 328768

Food For Thought

Between a third and a half of all cancers may be caused by eating the wrong foods. In this bestselling book Dr Coleman explains which foods to avoid and which to eat to reduce your risk of developing cancer. He also lists foods known to be associated with a wide range of other diseases including Asthma, Gall Bladder Disease, Headaches, Heart Trouble, High Blood Pressure, Indigestion and many more.

Years of research have gone into the writing of this book which explains the facts about mad cow disease, vegetarian eating, microwaves, drinking water, food poisoning, food irradiation and additives. It contains all the information you need about vitamins, carbohydrates, fats and proteins plus a list of superfoods which Dr Coleman believes can improve your health and protect you from a wide range of health problems. The book also includes a "slim-for-life" programme with 48 quick slimming tips to help you lose weight safely and permanently.

' ... *a guide to healthy eating which reads like a thriller*'
(The Good Book Guide)

'*Dr Vernon Coleman is one of our most enlightened, trenchant and sensible dispensers of medical advice*'
(The Observer)

paperback £12.95

Published by European Medical Journal
Order from Publishing House • Trinity Place • Barnstaple •
Devon EX32 9HJ • England
Telephone 01271 328892 • Fax 01271 328768